Oxford Medical Publications

Evidence for Population Health

Evidence for Population Health

Richard F. Heller
Professor of Public Health
Evidence for Population Health Unit
University of Manchester
Manchester
U.K.

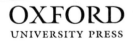

OXFORD
UNIVERSITY PRESS

*This book has been printed digitally and produced in a standard specification
in order to ensure its continuing availability*

OXFORD
UNIVERSITY PRESS

Great Clarendon Street, Oxford OX2 6DP
Oxford University Press is a department of the University of Oxford.
It furthers the University's objective of excellence in research, scholarship,
and education by publishing worldwide in
Oxford New York
Auckland Cape Town Dar es Salaam Hong Kong Karachi
Kuala Lumpur Madrid Melbourne Mexico City Nairobi
New Delhi Shanghai Taipei Toronto
With offices in
Argentina Austria Brazil Chile Czech Republic France Greece
Guatemala Hungary Italy Japan South Korea Poland Portugal
Singapore Switzerland Thailand Turkey Ukraine Vietnam

Oxford is a registered trade mark of Oxford University Press
in the UK and in certain other countries
Published in the United States
by Oxford University Press Inc., New York

ISBN 978-0-19-852974-3

Foreword

Stephen Leeder

Professor of Public Health and Community Medicine
at the University of Sydney

How do I know when I am passing a shop that sells expensive, fashionable clothes, even without judging their quality or appeal? The window displays carry no price tags! The absence of price tags sends a message that only extremely wealthy people should consider this fur coat, that silk dress, these crocodile-skin shoes.

Health is not a fashion commodity. It should not be available only to those with unlimited means who are unconcerned about price. Indeed, there is a strong argument that, when considering human rights, a right to health should be on the agenda. In any case, paying for better health and health care is increasingly a concern of government. As economies flourish, governments assume greater responsibility for health. A responsible government does not invest blindly in health. It does not go shopping in a fashion store for medical and hospital care where there are no price tags. Economic responsibility demands of government that it invest wisely and well.

One of the surprises that come to managers and administrators who move to the health portfolio with prior experience in commerce and industry is the paucity of price tags, and the dearth of dependable information that enables the health investor to know what he or she gets for their investment. Many countries struggle to identify accurately the causes of death of their citizens. What are the principal causes of illness, disability, and suffering in my community? How much illness does this, or that, exposure (say, cigarette smoking) cause in my country? If we modified that exposure, who would benefit? What would it cost to achieve this?

When a national budget is struck, a health minister needs numbers to put on the table, beside those from the education, industry, infrastructure, and defence portfolios, to mount his or her argument for resources. True, much community concern about health is satisfied if governments simply provide a service, irrespective of its quality. But to proceed on this basis alone is fraught with risk, and does nothing dependable to improve the health of the nation. Yes, the health minister should be able to argue his or her case using estimates of service cost, but also to supplement these estimates with information about the health gains he or she expects to follow from investment.

The book that follows seeks to provide ways whereby health managers and ministers can get information about the causes of illness, and the extent to which illness patterns can be attributed to particular causes, and the sections of the community where health service intervention will yield the best results. The text walks the reader through the steps they need to take. For readers with an interest in the mathematics of these calculations, the author provides details in the appendices. Health managers may wish to delegate these calculations, but must own the results to present to their colleagues when seeking public resources to provide better opportunities for health.

The book also teaches us that there is likely to be more useful information available to us than we first thought. This information comes in two forms—first, from published papers and reports from other places but with broad applicability, and second, from statistical collections that may lie gathering dust in government departments.

In my country, the latter is certainly true: in the past two decades, epidemiologists and managers have worked to convert these collections into useful information. One colleague, who had spent too long with death certificates, mordantly described this exercise as 'exhuming data cemeteries!' We often feel swamped with data while we starve for information. This book explains how to move from the swamp to high ground, and apply data to make the case for health investment, argue for preventive programs, assess the impact of new investments, and change track if something does not work. Most importantly, it gives hope to the health service manager that he or she can actually do measurable good. If you are a manager who wants to do good, this is a book that will help you to do good, or even better.

March 2005

Preface

The inspiration for this book comes from a career spanning clinical practice and public health teaching and research. I have attempted to make contributions to improvements in clinical care, both through my own clinical practice and through research into health care issues. A recent change of job and continent has allowed me to wonder what this effort has achieved. My efforts at clinical practice might have helped a few people, but I would have to struggle to show how my research has changed anything. I do think that I have made a contribution to the career development of a number of health professionals around the world, and through them maybe to others. By focusing on health care research, I will have missed the opportunity to be involved in the tackling of larger issues. While health care will help individuals feel better, its impact on the health of the population is less than that of major public health interventions. I have been so impressed with the benefits of evidence-based medicine, both on health care and on making health care workers think more clearly, that I want to extend this to public health. Many of the stimuli to the creation of evidence-based medicine are present in public health—such as the common use of anecdote rather than science in diagnosis and choice of intervention.

This book aims to show how developing and applying an evidence base to public health can help. Those of you who read it will understand why we need this evidence base, what are the philosophical underpinnings of the population approach, and what are the methods that we can use in evidence for population health. Some of these methods are well established, others are newly developed by my colleagues and myself. I hope that you, the reader, will apply these methods to your own thinking, research and practice.

The book is aimed at all those interested in a population approach to health. I have attempted to show what understanding is relevant at the student, practitioner and policy-making levels. I have attempted to include themes from international health, as well as from my own practice perspective in Australia and the UK, based on my experience with the International Clinical Epidemiology Network.

I have structured the book in three sections, to follow the 'Population Health Evidence Cycle', with which readers will become familiar. First, *Ask the question*—what is evidence for population health and why do we need it? Second, *Collect the evidence*—what measures can we make? Third, *Understand and use the evidence*—how can professionals and the public understand and use evidence to improve population health?

February 2005   RFH

Acknowledgements

I would like to thank my wife Ann for her tremendous help and encouragement, Steve Leeder for his painstaking editorial advice, Jacqueline Scholtz for her help in seeking copyright permissions, and Stewart Taylor for his help with the figures.

RFH, 2005

Contents

The book is organized in three sections. Each one follows the schema of the Population Health Evidence Cycle (described in Chapter 1). In order to develop an evidence base for population health, we need to **ask** the right question, **collect** appropriate data and calculate appropriate measures of population impact, then **understand** and **use** the data provided for population health policy-making.

Part I

Ask the question

What is the need for evidence for population health?

The first section of this book attempts to provide a theoretical rationale for both the concept of the population approach and the need to develop methods for the development and implementation of an evidence base.

Chapter 1

What is evidence for population health?

This chapter asks the question why we need to consider evidence for population health and how can it draw on the successes of evidence-based medicine?

The term 'evidence for population health' was coined in 2002, with the explicit aim of learning the lessons of evidence-based medicine (EBM) and applying them to the population setting.[1] EBM has had a major impact on clinical care throughout the world. It arose from the discipline of clinical epidemiology, a term which no one could understand, but which used the population sciences to research and then teach a scientific approach to clinical practice. What was missing from clinical epidemiology, and also from EBM, was a population focus. While the population sciences were central to the methods used, most practitioners were not thinking beyond the individual to the population. In fact, this criticism has also been applied to much epidemiological research, which has been based on identifying the predictors of health outcomes among individuals—we discuss the similar movement to bring the population back into epidemiology later, in Chapter 2.

> As improvements in public health are of major potential value, the academic public health community has a great need to develop a methodology of similar impact to that of EBM in the clinical arena to provide an evidence base for population as well as individual health problems. While there have been important advances in the population health sciences, these have not matched the developments and impact of EBM.[1]

Why was EBM so successful, and what lessons can we learn from it? What are the failures of EBM, and how can we do better with our population counterpart?

The success of EBM has been due to many things, but most important would be the central philosophy of providing a scientific basis to health care. There are two major themes to the way that EBM has come to be practiced—the 'statistical' or methods development and the 'implementation' or application of the methods.[1] It is the implementation end of EBM that has not developed as quickly or successfully as the statistical, and as we think evidence for population health, we must make sure that we focus clearly on how to ensure that evidence can be implemented to improve population health.

Why population and not public health?

Without getting into terminology debates, I have chosen to use 'population' rather than 'public' health. This emphasizes the contrast between the individual and the population, and ensures that if the speciality of public health reverts to previous terminology such as community medicine the central notion of the population will not be lost. Kindig and Stoddart have used the term population health, which they define as 'the health outcomes of a group of individuals, including the distribution of such outcomes within the group',[2] and they discuss a number of other definitions. Whatever the various definitions include, they do at least reinforce the use of the term population. Others have emphasized the importance of evidence in public health[3–6] and we are keen to relate evidence for population health to the current practice of public health. To help with this link, we have made our own definition to show public health practitioners that evidence and the population health sciences are central to what they do (or should do).

Public health is defined as 'Use of theory, experience and evidence derived through the population sciences to improve the Health of the community, in a way that best meets the implicit and explicit needs of that community (the Public).'[7]

To emphasize the importance of evidence to public health practice, the Population Health Evidence Cycle[8] can be used, and we have organized the content of this book using this basic structure.

Figure 1.1 could be drawn in the shape of a spiral rather than a cycle, to reflect the fact that this is a continuing saga, where finding an

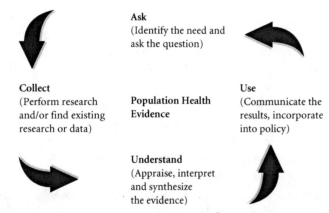

Fig. 1.1 The Population Health Evidence cycle[8].

Based on and reprinted from the coursework of the MPHe, University of Manchester, http://www.mphe.man.ac.uk

answer to one question will raise even more questions. Even the simplest question, if it leads to data collection and eventual use in health policy decisions, will require an evaluation of the policy which takes us round the cycle again. This of course, is based on Popper's approach of the scientific method[9]—not an accident, as I am keen to emphasize that we are dealing with science and that population sciences are just as much science as any other.

Why do we need an evidence-based approach in population health?

Different countries have developed the practice of public health in different ways, but each population requires some professional group or groups to take responsibility for maintaining and dealing with threats to its health. As with clinical practice, public health practice can provide numerous examples of activities which were introduced with the best of intentions but which were later found not to be worthwhile. Many of the community-based health promotion interventions, which are the mainstay of public health practice, have been found to be ineffective (or even harmful) when subjected to the rigours of the randomized controlled trial.[10–14] Lung cancer and multiphasic screening programmes have usually been found to be ineffective (although newer technologies are being tried again for lung cancer). The current practice of public health, which includes health promotion, is full of examples of interventions which have either been shown previously to be ineffective, have not been evaluated and are not going to be, or are aimed at an unachievable target. The UK government has set targets for reducing health inequalities which include those that are not achievable—reflecting an inadequate understanding of the methodologies to be described in later chapters. There is thus a need not only to develop an evidence base, so that ineffective interventions are not introduced or continued, but also to make sure that policy-makers are aware of some of the requirements of the rules of evidence.

Key summary points

+ *The Student.* The population health evidence cycle describes an organizing format for thinking about how to incorporate evidence into public health practice.

+ *The Practitioner.* The similarities between evidence-based medicine and evidence for population health allow us to consider both 'statistical' and 'implementational' methods to develop and incorporate an evidence base into public health.

+ *The Policy-maker.* Reflections on how EBM has changed the face of clinical decision-making should help implement evidence into public health policy-making.

References

1   Heller R. F. and Page J. H. A population perspective to evidence based medicine: 'evidence for population health'. *Journal of Epidemiology and Community Health* 2002; **56**: 45–7.

2   Kindig D. and Stoddart G. What is population health? *Am. J. Public Health* 2003; **93**: 380–3.

3   Muir Gray J. A. *Evidence-Based Health Care.* Edinburgh: Churchill Livingstone, 2001.

4   Glasziou P. and Longbottom H. Evidence-based public health practice. *Aust. N. Z. J. Public Health* 1999; **23**: 436–40.

5   Gray J. A. Evidence-based public health–what level of competence is required? *J. Public Health Med.* 1997; **19**: 65–8.

6 Brownson R. C. *Evidence-based Public Health.* Oxford: Oxford University Press, 2003.

7 Heller R. F., Heller T. D., Pattison S. Putting the public back into public health. Part I. A re-definition of public health. *Public Health* 2003; **117**: 62–5.

8 Heller R. F., Heller T. D., Pattison S. Putting the public back into public health. Part II. How can public health be accountable to the public? *Public Health* 2003; **117**: 66–71.

9 Popper K. *The Logic of Scientific Discovery* (translation of *Logik der Forschung*). London: Hutchinson, 1959.

10 Merzel C. and D'Afflitti J. Reconsidering community-based health promotion: promise, performance, and potential. *Am. J. Public Health* 2003; **93**: 557–74.

11 Ebrahim S. and Smith G. D. Systematic review of randomised controlled trials of multiple risk factor interventions for preventing coronary heart disease. *BMJ* 1997; **314**: 1666–74.

12 Ebrahim S. and Smith G. D. Effects of the Heartbeat Wales programme. Effects of government policies on health behaviour must be studied. *BMJ* 1998; **317**: 886.

13 Bauman K. E., Suchindran C. M., Murray D. M. The paucity of effects in community trials: is secular trend the culprit? *Prev. Med.* 1999; **28**: 426–9.

14 Hallfors D., Cho H., Livert D., Kadushin C. Fighting back against substance abuse: are community coalitions winning? *Am. J. Prev. Med.* 2002; **23**: 237–45.

Chapter 2

The population or the individual in public health?

This chapter explains that there are special influences on health from the 'context' in which we live, beyond the genetic and behavioural make-up of individuals.

The genetic make-up of individuals, and their behaviour, both contribute to the chance that a particular disease will develop. Many modern day research findings have identified the relationship between individual variables and health outcomes. There are, however, other factors at work. The environment produces influences on the individual, through exposure to communicable disease organisms and chemical and other agents. Beyond these individual exposures, which to some extent can be avoided by behaviour change, there are other factors which influence health more extensively than any of these. These are population causes of disease. If you had lived 100 years ago, you would have had a much shorter life expectancy than you have today, despite a similar genetic make-up and possibly similar individual behaviour patterns. If you live in Africa, you have a vastly different life expectancy than if you live in Europe, and the variations within Africa and Europe are as large or larger than the differences between the continents. These big between-population differences over time and geography are unlikely to be explained by genetic factors or by individual behaviour patterns. There are large 'population' or 'contextual' (i.e. the context in which individuals live and behave) influences on health.

Epidemiologists have been accused of focusing their research attention too much on the causes of disease in individuals. 'Risk factor epidemiology' has used the research methods of the population health sciences to predict disease outcomes among individuals, to reflect their behaviour or characteristics. Predicting the development of heart disease by knowledge of blood cholesterol, blood pressure, cigarette smoking and other characteristics is an excellent example of this, and has underpinned efforts to prevent heart disease which have been applied with considerable success.

The human genome project has more recently identified the genetic variability of the human species. This is leading to a resurgence of genetic epidemiology, where epidemiologists are setting up research programmes to link the newly discovered genetic markers of an individual's genome to disease outcomes.

In all this, although population sciences have been used, and the findings have been (or in the case of genetic epidemiology will be) of help to improve public health, the impact of the population in which individuals exist have largely been ignored. This criticism applies to much of current epidemiological research, and to the practice of public health. There is now a move to 'bring the population back into epidemiology and public health'.

Some landmark articles in the *American Journal of Public Health* in 1996 produced a wake-up call to epidemiologists. Susser[1,2] identified the need for 'eco-epidemiology' and Pearce made a plea for a rediscovery of the population perspective.[3] McMichael later indicated the importance of large-scale social and environmental change on health.[4]

Let's take the example of risks of heart disease. Levels of cigarette smoking, blood cholesterol, blood pressure and obesity (amongst other factors) predict the risk that an individual runs of developing both non-fatal and fatal heart attacks. But what determines the individuals' levels of these factors? Some genetic factors are involved, and there are individual behaviour patterns. There are wider societal determinants of behaviour, which must not be ignored if we are to understand why people smoke and eat high fat and high salt foods and to reduce exposure to these factors. Table 2.1 shows how those living in deprived neighbourhoods are more likely to have cardiovascular disease risk factors present than others. Individual characteristics operate within a powerful population context that may be a strong predictor of disease at the population level.[5]

A number of neighbourhood and environmental influences have been found to influence mortality.[6] A review of 25 studies has found that in all but two, there was a statistically significant association

Table 2.1 Odds ratio (with 95% confidence intervals) for the presence of three risk factors in those exposed to neighbourhood deprivation, having adjusted for the individual factors of sex, age and education (n = 9240)[14]

Presence of risk factor in individual	Odds ratio from living in low part (bottom 16%) of the distribution of social status of neighbourhood environment
Current smoking	1.69 (1.42–2.01)
No physical activity	1.61 (1.34–1.93)
Obesity	1.18 (1.02–1.36)

between at least one measure of social environment and a health outcome after adjusting for individual level socio-economic status.[7] While there is a clear need to examine the wider population influences on health, the final determinants of health outcomes are going to include population (or contextual) and individual level variables, and where possible analysis should include both.[8,9]

The Ecological Fallacy

Ecological studies (where area or population level variables alone are examined to see if they explain health outcomes) have been regarded as low-level evidence by the epidemiological community. The Ecological Fallacy describes the problem which can occur when inferences are made about individuals based on aggregate data for a group. However, Pearce has shown that we should not ignore ecological studies,[9] and as we will discuss later when reviewing the hierarchy of evidence required for public health decision-making, we will not place these studies as low in the hierarchy as others have done.

Geoffrey Rose and the population approach

One of the most important contributions to the theoretical framework of public health comes from Geoffrey Rose. Geoffrey was a clinical epidemiologist who was able to articulate the difference between the impact of individual and population causes of disease. His paper 'Sick individuals and sick populations'[10] has become a very important landmark in attempts to improve public health. The paper was reprinted in 2001[11] (together with a number of commentaries[12]), and makes a number of key points. The first, is that the determinants of disease in individuals *within* a population can be distinct from the determinants of variation in disease rate *between* populations. In other words, risk factors acting at the population level may affect the rate of disease in a population and this is different from the predictors of disease among individuals. For example, the question as to why some people develop hypertension is a different question from why do some populations have much hypertension, whilst in others it is rare. Rose also points out that investigations of factors associated with causation of conditions in individuals using conventional case control methods will fail to identify risk factors for which there is insufficient variation in exposure within the study population. In such cases, clues about underlying causal factors must be sought from comparing exposures in populations with different rates of disease. For example, the contribution of diet to the causation of cardiovascular disease is more evident when comparing populations in different countries than when comparing individuals within a country. For other factors there may be sufficient variation among individuals within populations to identify potential causative relationships. Smoking and genetic inheritance have been identified as potential causes of cardiovascular disease using individual data within countries. However, information from both levels of aggregation is often needed to identify potential causes of disease and formulate appropriate health care responses.

The next point that Geoffrey Rose makes is that it is important to consider both the 'population' and 'high-risk' approaches to prevention. He also coined the term 'Prevention Paradox'. This means that a population based intervention, while being an important strategy, will require many people to change and few to benefit. (The converse is the 'Treatment Paradox', where the apparent benefit to the individual seen by the clinician and a grateful patient may not translate into much benefit for the population[13].) There is a risk that policy-makers may be unduly influenced by these paradoxes, and follow policies aimed at individuals who can be seen to benefit rather than at the greater population need. These concepts underlie the need for appropriate measures of population impact—to which we return in Chapter 4.

Conclusion

There are important theoretical reasons for thinking in population terms, and they reinforce the call to 'bring the population back into epidemiology and public health'!

Key summary points

- *The Student.* There are both individual (genetic and behavioural) and population (contextual) causes of disease, which are distinct.

- *The Practitioner.* The population (contextual) influences on health should not be ignored in attempts to understand disease causation.

- *The Policy-maker.* The prevention paradox (many have to change for few to benefit) and the treatment paradox (benefits to individual patients may not translate to much population benefit) are important—health policy should not take undue note of influences relating to individuals.

References

1 Susser M. and Susser E. Choosing a future for epidemiology: I. Eras and paradigms. *Am. J. Public Health* 1996; **86**: 668–73.

2 Susser M. and Susser E. Choosing a future for epidemiology: II. From black box to Chinese boxes and eco-epidemiology. *Am. J. Public Health* 1996; **86**: 674–7.

3 Pearce N. Traditional epidemiology, modern epidemiology, and public health. *Am. J. Public Health* 1996; **86**: 678–83.

4 McMichael A. J. Prisoners of the proximate: loosening the constraints on epidemiology in an age of change. *Am. J. Epidemiol.* 1999; **149**: 887–97.

5 Pearce N. The ecological fallacy strikes back. *J. Epidemiol. Community Health* 2000; **54**: 326–7.

6 Yen I. H. and Kaplan G. A. Neighborhood social environment and risk of death: multilevel evidence from the Alameda County Study. *Am. J. Epidemiol.* 1999; **149**: 898–907.

7 Pickett K. E. and Pearl M. Multilevel analyses of neighbourhood socioeconomic context and health outcomes: a critical review. *J. Epidemiol. Community Health* 2001; **55**: 111–22.

8 Diez-Roux A. V. Bringing context back into epidemiology: variables and fallacies in multilevel analysis. *Am. J. Public Health* 1998; **88**: 216–22.

9 Pearce N. Epidemiology as a population science. *Int. J. Epidemiol.* 1999; **28**: S1015–18.

10 Rose G. Sick individuals and sick populations. *Int. J. Epidemiol.* 1985; **14**: 32–8.

11 Rose G. Sick individuals and sick populations. *Int. J. Epidemiol.* 2001; **30**: 427–32.

12 Ebrahim S. Commentary: Sick populations and sick individuals. *Int. J. Epidemiol.* 2001; **30**: 433–4.

13 Hersh A. L., Black W. C., Tosteson A. N. Estimating the population impact of an intervention: a decision-analytic approach. *Stat. Methods Med. Res.* 1999; **8**: 311–30.

14 Sundquist J., Malmstrom M., Johansson S. E. Cardiovascular risk factors and the neighbourhood environment: a multilevel analysis. *Int. J. Epidemiol.* 1999; **28**: 841–5.

Chapter 3

Shifting the distribution

This chapter shows that shifting the distribution of a variable for the whole population is an important concept, which adds to considerations of reducing risk factors in individuals and underlies the population approach to health improvement.

One of the major implications of the population causes of disease is that you may produce a larger health benefit by tackling issues at a population rather than at an individual level. The theoretical reasons for this have again been outlined by Geoffrey Rose, who discussed the benefits of the population approach to reducing risk and contrasted it with the high-risk approach,[1] as we have seen in Chapter 2. The discussion goes something like this:

Most biological variables are 'normally' distributed in the population. A variable such as blood pressure increases with age, and thus the distribution will be skewed according to the age distribution of the population in which it is being examined. Blood pressure is a good example, as there is a clinical definition of high blood pressure. Let's define 'hypertension' as a systolic BP of 140 mmHg or more. If the BP distribution shown in Figure 3.1 is as in the continuous line (London civil servants), a higher proportion of the population will be defined as having hypertension than if the distribution is as in the dotted line (Kenyan nomads). If we could shift the distribution from that in the continuous line to that in the dotted line, we could reduce the proportion of the population who have hypertension.

A similar pattern can be seen for geographic influences on Body Mass Index (BMI, which is weight/height^2, a measure of obesity). The graph in Figure 3.2 is drawn from data on samples of men aged 40–59 years in seven Asian and five Latin American centres from the International Clinical Epidemiology Network (INCLEN).[2] We see

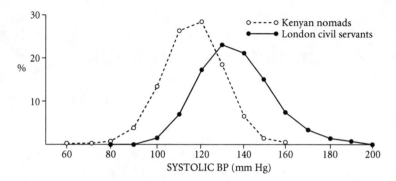

Fig. 3.1 Distribution of systolic blood pressure in Kenya and London.[1]

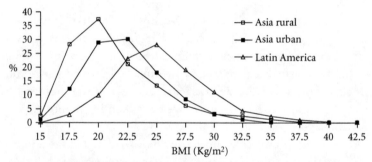

Fig. 3.2 Distribution of age-adjusted body mass index (BMI) in Asian and Latin American urban and rural men.[2]

that as we go from rural Asian populations, through urban Asian populations to more industrialized Latin American populations, the distribution of BMI shifts to the right.

As with the hypertension example above, you can see that shifting the whole distribution of the Latin American and urban Asian population samples towards the left, as represented by the rural Asian populations, would reduce the prevalence of overweight and obesity as well as the population mean BMI. If we consider definitions of 'overweight' and 'obesity' as a BMI of 25 and 30 respectively, we can see that shifting the distribution from that of Latin American to Asian men will reduce the prevalence of overweight from over 25 per cent to less than 20 per cent (urban) or less than 15 per cent (rural). It will reduce the prevalence of obesity from over 10 per cent in Latin American men to less than 5 per cent in Asian men in our samples.

Back to Geoffrey Rose again, who wrote a paper 'The population mean predicts the number of deviant individuals'.[3] The paper considers deviants as those whose level of hypertension, alcohol intake and BMI have deviated far enough from the population mean towards the extremes of the distribution to make them clinical 'cases'. The paper concludes:

> These findings imply that distributions of health related characteristics move up and down as a whole: the frequency of 'cases' can be understood only in the context of a population's characteristics. The population thus carries a collective responsibility for its own health and well-being, including that of its deviants.[3]

A hypothetical example of the population approach to blood pressure reduction

The example in Table 3.1 uses data from a large population of 422,594 people.[4] There were 4856 CHD events (fatal and non-fatal) over 10 years. Columns 2 and 3 show the distribution of various categories of blood pressure and the risk of subsequent CHD events. The last column is one example of a hypothetical change if we could shift the blood pressure distribution within the population downwards (thus relatively more people would be 'exposed' to lower blood pressure levels and relatively fewer 'exposed' to high levels). The shift of 5 per cent we have used for illustration purposes could perhaps be produced by a reduction in obesity or salt intake across the population.

When we make the calculations, we see that the numbers of CHD deaths in the population would be reduced from 4856 to 4783. Thus, even a small shift in the distribution of blood pressure within the population could lead to a demonstrable reduction in outcomes. You might want to calculate the impact of other strategies—such as reduction in risk of the highest blood pressure category to that in the category below (i.e. a high-risk strategy). This is a hypothetical example, but illustrates the potential of a population approach.

Table 3.1 Shifting the blood pressure distribution

Diastolic BP category	Observed risk of CHD events over 10 years per 1000 people	True population distribution 1	Number of CHD events*	Hypothetical population distribution 2 (shifted down by 5% from each category to the lower one)	Number of CHD events*
< 70 mmHg	6.4	30119	193	39981	256
70–79 mmHg	7.4	112186	830	111726	827
80–89 mmHg	10.2	160695	1639	155546	1587
90–99 mmHg	14.7	85056	1250	82170	1208
100–109 mmHg	22.6	27340	618	26333	595
110+ mmHg	45.3	7198	326	6838	310
Total		422594	4856	422594	4783

* Number of events calculated by applying risk to the population in the column before it

Table 3.2 Possible effects on coronary heart disease by changes in cholesterol levels

Simulation	Percentage reduction in CHD cases or deaths
All reduce their cholesterol level to less than 5.0 mmol/l	53.4
Those in the highest cholesterol group (over 7.8 mmol/l) reduce their cholesterol level to 6.5–7.8 mmol/l	2.0
Everyone shifts down a category	25.9
Everyone reduces cholesterol to less than 6.5 mmol/l	11.1
Everyone reduces cholesterol by 0.6 mmol/l	9.2
Everyone reduces cholesterol by 0.3 mmol/l	4.8

Note: we return to this example in Chapter 4, Table 4.3.

From McPherson et al.[5]

Another example is provided for the possible effects on coronary heart disease by changes in cholesterol levels.[5] This is based on a review of the relative risk from cholesterol levels of 5.2–6.5 mmol/l, 6.5–7.8 mmol/l and over 7.8 mmol/l of developing CHD of 1.75, 2.57 and 3.46 (relative to levels below 5.2 mmol/l) and prevalences of these levels of 41 per cent, 21 per cent and 7 per cent. Table 3.2 shows McPherson and colleagues' estimate of the possible effects on CHD following changes in cholesterol levels.

Reducing health inequalities—close the gap or shift the distribution?

The lessons of Geoffrey Rose, and the concept of shifting the distribution, have been forgotten in recent years by many health policy makers. An important example is in the field of health inequalities.

The Department of Health in the UK has decided to attempt to reduce health inequalities (see Chapter 5—Evaluating population-based interventions). One of the spurs to attempting this is the repeated demonstration of a widening gap in health outcomes between the extremes of the social distribution. A government programme, Tackling Health Inequalities, has identified two main targets, which are to close the gap between those at the lowest end of the social spectrum and the population as a whole (for infant mortality and life expectancy) http://www.dh.gov.uk/assetRoot/04/01/93/62/04019362.pdf. There is a fundamental debate as to whether 'closing the gap' is the appropriate goal or whether it is more appropriate to attempt to improve the health of the whole population. As the following example shows, it is probably impossible to close the gap since the widening gap is itself a function of the changing demographic composition of the population—upward mobility.

In recent years, the health of all groups has improved, although the gap between the extremes of the social distribution has increased. In 1971, 25.5 per cent of UK men were classified as social class I or II (professional/managerial) and 24.8 per cent as social class IV or V (partly skilled/unskilled). By 1991, this had changed to 37.8 per cent and 19.7 per cent respectively. Those left behind have worse health than those who ascend the social scale, so unless some adjustment is made for the fact that over time those in social classes IV/V represent a different proportion of the population and a proportion expected to have poor health, just comparing trends between social classes over time will give a misleading picture of apparently widening divisions in health between the social extremes. Hence, as the health and the living standards of the whole population improve and the population becomes upwardly mobile, the gap will widen. This is a consequence of demographic change, and once this is understood it should help ensure that inappropriate attempts to close a gap that cannot be closed will cease.

One example of this is a paper in the *BMJ* which shows that as a consequence of upward mobility of the population, population mortality from cardiovascular disease has declined.[6] Upward mobility between 1971 and 1991 accounted on its own for 18 per cent of the decline in cardiovascular disease deaths seen in the UK over that time period. Thus shifting the distribution is likely to be a more appropriate intervention than closing the gap.

Should we look at social differences or the health of the whole population?

Rawls developed the 'minimax' or 'difference' principle. He says that provided the poor get richer as a result of change, it does not matter if the gap between the rich and the poor increases: however, economic and social advantages for the better-off members of a society are only justified if they benefit the worst-off.[7]

Our population approach is consistent with Rawls' theory, and suggests to policy-makers that as well as looking at equity issues within a population, we should be examining the impact of any health policy on the population as a whole, not being surprised if the social divide appears to increase.

Despite this debate, there is no doubt that attempts to improve the health of the worst-off within any population, and the worst-off between populations should be a key part of health policy.

Some suggestions have been made that the level of inequalities within a population determines the level of health of the whole population—if this were true it would provide justification for a reduction in within-population inequalities. A systematic review of the literature, however, provides 'little support for a direct effect of income inequality on health per se'.[8]

Key summary points

- *The Student.* Shifting the population distribution of a characteristic will also impact on the proportion of individuals at the extremes, and provides the rationale for population-wide interventions.

- *The Practitioner.* Shifting the population distribution of a characteristic will also impact on the proportion of individuals at the extremes, thus reducing the numbers of people eligible for treatment.

- *The Policy-maker.* Health policies aimed at closing the inequalities gap between the extremes of a population distribution are based on flawed logic. Health policy should focus on shifting the population distribution, and on the lowest groups within in a population.

References

1 Rose G. Sick individuals and sick populations. *Int. J. Epidemiol.* 2001; **30**: 427–32.

2 Body mass index and cardiovascular disease risk factors in seven Asian and five Latin American centers: data from the International Clinical Epidemiology Network (INCLEN). *Obes. Res.* 1996; **4**: 221–8.

3 Rose G. and Day S. The population mean predicts the number of deviant individuals. *BMJ* 1990; **301**: 1031–4.

4 MacMahon S., Peto R., Cutler J., Collins R., Sorlie P., Neaton J. *et al.* Blood pressure, stroke, and coronary heart disease. Part 1, Prolonged differences in blood pressure: prospective observational studies corrected for the regression dilution bias. *Lancet* 1990; **335**: 765–74.

5 McPherson K., Britton A., Causer L. *Coronary Heart Disease. Estimating the impact of changes in risk factors.* London: The Stationery Office: National Heart Forum, 2002.

6 Heller R. F., McElduff P., Edwards R. Impact of upward social mobility on population mortality: analysis with routine data. *BMJ* 2002; **325**: 134.

7 Rawls J. *A Theory of Justice.* Oxford: Clarendon Press, 1972.

8 Lynch J., Smith G. D., Harper S., Hillemeier M., Ross N., Kaplan G. A. *et al.* Is income inequality a determinant of population health? Part 1. A systematic review. *Milbank Q.* 2004; **82**: 5–99.

Part II

Collect the evidence
What measures should we make?

The second section of the book is devoted to the
second stage of the Population Evidence Cycle—collect
the evidence. The main measures discussed are the
population impact measures with which I have been
working and which offer a different approach to the
measurement of the disease burden. They are explained
and set in the context of more traditional measures of
risk, benefit and disease burden. Chapters on which
outcome measure to use, how the evidence hierarchy
could be developed to reflect a population approach
and the role of health informatics in data collection
complete the section.

Chapter 4

Measuring the population impact

This chapter reports on a number of ways of examining the impact of risk factors and of intervention benefits on the population as a whole. We begin with the most recent of these measures, population impact measures, and then reflect on the measures which have been in use for a longer time.

Measuring the population impact of risk

Only a subset of the total population will be at risk from a particular exposure (for example, a group defined by age, gender or ethnicity), and only a proportion of those exposed will have become cases as a result of their exposure, as will a (smaller) proportion of those not exposed. Figure 4.1 shows the interplay between the population, exposure to a risk factor and the occurrence of disease (cases). The small black box represents those who have become cases due to their exposure.

The figure is not drawn to scale: in fact the relative sizes of each box will be different for different diseases in different populations. You can see that you can easily calculate the ratio of each box to the others.

Let's review the traditional measures of risk and how they can be understood from this figure.

The ratio of the occurrence of cases in the exposed and non-exposed parts of the population at risk can tell us something about the risk of exposure to becoming a case.

Using a cohort study, we would take a sample of the population at risk, some exposed to the risk factor and some not exposed. We then follow all of them over time, during which cases will occur among the exposed and the non-exposed. The ratio of these

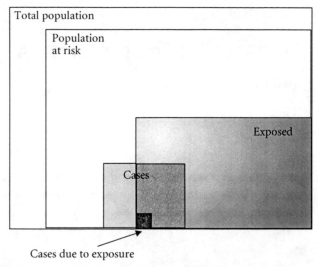

Cases due to exposure

Fig. 4.1 Cases due to exposure are seen in the context of the total number of cases, the total number exposed, the population at risk of exposure and the whole population. This information comes from case-control and cohort studies, and the components are used to derive the various measures of risk described in the text. (Redrawn from[3].)

is the relative risk (RR), which is the incidence (rate of occurrence of new cases) in the exposed, divided by the incidence of cases in the non-exposed.

Using a case control study, we would identify some of the cases and some of the non-cases (controls), and examine their prior exposure to the possible risk factor. The measure of the effect of exposure is expressed as an odds ratio (OR) which is the ratio of the odds of having been exposed if you are a case, to the odds of having been exposed if you are a non-case. In many situations (where the frequency of exposure is low in the population), the odds ratio can be used as a proxy for the relative risk. I suggest you look at standard epidemiology texts for more detail on this, and a more traditional way of measuring these risks.[1]

The population perspective

The RR and OR only require information from a part of the figure—those who are exposed, and those who are not exposed. The rest of the population is not included. Being consistent with our mission of extending from the individual to the population, we now need to examine the impact of exposure on the whole population, not just the individuals who may have been exposed to the risk factor.

Traditional approaches

Epidemiological measures of population risk   The idea of attempting to extend measures of risk from epidemiological studies to the population is not new. Levin first made an estimate of the amount of lung cancer in a population of men that could be attributed to cigarette smoking,[2] and the measure he described is now called the population attributable risk (PAR). This concept has subsequently collected different versions, names and meanings, which have made it difficult to understand and use. The population attributable risk proportion (PAR or PARP or PAF or PAR%: PAR for simplicity) refers to the proportion of the population's risk that would be removed if the risk factor was abolished. It is derived from two measures: the first is the RR, which is derived from a cohort study, or estimated (as OR) from a case-control study, as described in the section above. Then in calculating PAR we take into account the proportion of the population exposed to the risk factor. The details of the calculation are in Appendix A at the end of this chaper. We can describe the impact of risk on the population in a different way, producing a number of people who would have to be exposed in order to 'produce' one 'case' with the outcome of interest. This is very simply the reciprocal of the PAR, which is called the case impact number (CIN) and defined as the number of people with the disease for whom one case is attributable to the exposure.[3] It is one of the new population impact measures, others of which I describe more fully below.

An example of the use of PAR and CIN is seen in Table 4.1 (taken from reference[3]—data from reference[4]). Assume that the relative risk of coronary heart disease (CHD) and lung cancer from smoking is 1.62 and 14 respectively and that 30 per cent of the population are cigarette smokers.

Thus, 16 per cent and 80 per cent of the population burden of CHD and lung cancer respectively are due to cigarette smoking. Among every 638 cases of CHD, 100 are due to smoking, as are 100 among every 126 cases of lung cancer.

Table 4.1 Population attributable risk and case impact number—smoking and coronary heart disease and lung cancer

	Coronary heart disease	Lung cancer
Proportion of the disease in the population due to cigarette smoking: Population attributable risk (PAR)	0.157	0.796
Number of people with the disease for whom one case is attributable to the exposure: Case impact number (CIN)	6.38	1.26

Population impact measures

In order to extend the previously described measures of population disease burden, another set of measures is under development. They are designed for ease of communication to inform health policy[5] and are useful when examining both cause of disease (risk) and the benefits of interventions. Cause is considered in this section.

The measures add the incidence in the total population to the traditional measures of risk described above, as well as identifying a population base to which the results can be directly referred. However, they still include the measures used in the PAR. PAR can be calculated without knowing the baseline risk in the population, it gives a proportion (or percentage), and does not provide an absolute measure of rates or numbers affected. Our new measure is defined as 'the potential number of disease events prevented in your population over the next t years by eliminating a risk factor', and is called the 'Population Impact Number of Eliminating a Risk Factor (PIN-ER-t). Its calculation is in Appendix B at the end of this chapter.

An example

This example is taken from reference.[6] What is the impact of different levels of blood cholesterol on deaths from CHD in the population? We have known for a long time that although the relative risk of CHD increases with each increase in blood cholesterol category, there are fewer people at risk at higher cholesterol levels. Taking CHD death rates and applying to the distribution of blood cholesterol and the RR data from best available evidence[7] shows that 13 per cent of all CHD deaths in women are attributed to cholesterol levels of 7.8 mmol/l or more (PAR). The PAR is 18 per cent in those with lower cholesterol levels of 6.5–7.8 mmol/l and 16 per cent among those with levels of 5.5–6.5 mmol/l. Supposing we were doing this calculation in an average UK General Practice population of 10,000 people, we would find that the numbers of CHD deaths among women due to blood cholesterol are 0.88, 1.23, and 1.04 in those with levels of 7.8+, 6.5–7.8 and 5.5–6.5 respectively over three years (see Tables 4.2 and 4.3).

The surprises here are first the greater impact on the *population* occurs among the many with intermediate levels of blood cholesterol and second the somewhat low numbers of people who will actually die as a result of their cholesterol levels. I have shown the figures for women rather than men, where absolute risk is greater although the same gradients and implications for the population impact measures are seen.

Note: Expressing the PAR as the case impact number (CIN) shows that to produce one 'case' of CHD death, 7.7 women would be exposed to a cholesterol level of 7.8 mmol/l or more while only 5.6 would be exposed to the lower level of 6.5–7.8 mmol/l to produce one 'case' of CHD death.

The PAR is quite frequently used, although there is confusion over what it means and there are so many different formulations and

Table 4.2 Risk of death from coronary heart disease at different baseline cholesterol levels

	Cholesterol level	Relative risk associated with cholesterol level	Prevalence of cholesterol level in population [P_e]	Population attributable risk
Women aged <75 years	High blood cholesterol 7.8+ mmol/l	3.46	0.1	0.13
	Moderate blood cholesterol 6.5–7.8 mmol/l	2.57	0.22	0.18
	Above average blood cholesterol 5.2–6.5 mmol/l	1.75	0.39	0.16

Table 4.3 Risk of death from coronary heart disease at different baseline cholesterol levels: adding baseline risk and the population impact

Population	Cholesterol level	Relative risk associated with cholesterol level	Prevalence of cholesterol level in population [P_e]	Population Attributable Risk (PAR)	Numbers of deaths in 3 years prevented by eliminating risk factor (PIN-ER-3)*
Women age <75 (4591 women 3-year incidence of death 146.4/100,000 = 6.72 deaths expected in next 3 years)	High blood cholesterol 7.8+ mmol/l	3.46	0.1	0.13	0.88
	Moderate blood cholesterol 6.5–7.8 mmol/l	2.57	0.22	0.18	1.23
	Above average blood cholesterol 5.2–6.5 mmol/l	1.75	0.39	0.16	1.04

*Population Impact Number of Eliminating a Risk factor over 3 years.

expressions. I hope that the PIN-ER-*t* will now begin to find its place in the literature, and more importantly will be in common use amongst public health practitioners who wish to describe the impact of various risk factors on their populations. A number of methodological issues remain to be resolved, such as how to look at combinations of risk factors. We have also described the method for confidence intervals, and these can be found on a web site—http://simph.man.ac.uk/pinert

As you can see, there is much choice in which measure to use— maybe it is up to each person to pick the right measure for the right time, audience and purpose.

Measuring the population impact of interventions

Population impact of interventions: extending the number needed to treat to the population

The notion of using numbers related to the population at risk and the incidence of the health outcome in order to express the population impact is not new[8,9]. The impetus for their recent development came from the success that the 'number needed to treat' (NNT) statistic[10] has had. This is defined as the number of people who have to be treated to prevent one event. It has been enthusiastically adopted by the clinical community, who have found it very useful in clinical decision-making and in explaining risks and benefits to patients. It is easy to calculate, as the reciprocal of the absolute risk reduction $(I_e—I_u)$ where I_e is the incidence in those exposed to an intervention and I_u is the incidence in the unexposed.

The extension of the NNT to a population base requires an estimate of the proportion of the population with the disease or condition of interest, as well as the proportion of those with the disease who are eligible for and compliant with the intervention. Two statistics are defined as follows: the disease impact number (DIN) is defined as 'the number of those with the disease in question among whom one event will be prevented by the intervention'. The population impact number (PIN) is defined as 'the number of those in the whole population among whom one event will be prevented by the intervention'.

Figure 4.2 provides a graphic demonstration of the measures in a comparable way to Figure 4.1.

Extensions of the NNT to the population are designed to show the impact of an intervention on the population as a whole. If a highly efficacious intervention (that is, it strongly reduces risk or alleviates disease among those treated) can only be applied to a small proportion of the population, it may have less impact on the population as a whole than an intervention which does less for an individual but which can be applied to a greater proportion of the population. A good example is the use of thrombolysis in the treatment of stroke. This treatment works by restoring the blood supply to the brain. The efficacy is high, but only a small proportion of those who have a stroke can benefit as the trials show benefit only within the first three hours after the onset of the stroke, during which time the patient has to get to the hospital and have investigations to exclude a cerebral haemorrhage (which could be worsened by the treatment). The table

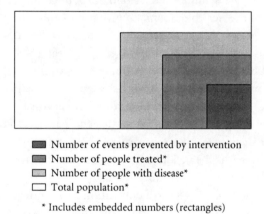

▓ Number of events prevented by intervention
▓ Number of people treated*
▢ Number of people with disease*
☐ Total population*

* Includes embedded numbers (rectangles)

Fig. 4.2 From Number Needed to Treat to the Population Impact. The people who can be treated with a particular intervention are a subgroup of those with the condition of interest, who themselves are a subset of the whole population. Number Needed to Treat (NNT) relates events prevented to those actually given treatment. Disease Impact Number (DIN) relates events prevented to the total with disease. Population Impact Number (PIN) relates events prevented to the total population. (From[28].)

below shows how it is possible to combine the results of the RRR of different interventions with the proportion of the population who will be able to be exposed to the treatment in producing a PIN and a DIN.

Suppose you were in charge of a population of around 120,000 people. If you introduced thrombolysis (expensive; must be given in 3 hours; cannot be given unless the patient has a clot) you could prevent one adverse health outcome (death or disability) in a year. If you introduced an organized stroke unit you could prevent six such events. These data, in combination with cost information about the two interventions, can then be fed into policy deliberations.

The example overleaf shows how a similar treatment for heart attack has a much greater population impact at older ages. Here, should we want to make policy decisions on eligibility for treatment at different ages, we would require more data such as how we can determine the value of a life saved at different ages. This type of decision-making is unlikely in reality, and it is more realistic that this information would be used to ensure that the elderly *do* get treated with effective interventions, and not ignored as a group. A number of studies have shown age and gender variations in treatment of heart disease.[11]

Table 4.4 Benefits of different proved interventions for treatment of non-haemorrhagic first stroke on basis of death or dependency at six months[5]

	Aspirin	Warfarin	Organised stroke unit	Thrombolysis
Absolute risk reduction	0.031	0.042	0.050	0.159
Proportion of stroke population treated[†]	0.70	0.29	0.70	0.04
Number needed to treat	33	24	20	7
Disease impact number	46	83	29	158
Population impact number	35450	63160	21980	120950

[†] Will vary according to economic and geographic setting.

Table 4.5 Benefits of thrombolysis after acute myocardial infarction by age for men in Australia on basis of deaths from days 0–35[5]

	Age (years)		
	<55	55–64	65–74
Absolute risk reduction	0.011	0.018	0.027
Proportion of population with acute myocardial infarction eligible for treatment*	0.54	0.49	0.40
Event rate of acute myocardial infarction per 100 000[†]	137	760	1523
Number needed to treat	91	56	37
Disease impact number	169	113	93
Population impact number	123000	14900	6100

* Assumes 77%, 70%, and 66% of patients in each ascending age group are admitted to hospital (due to deaths occurring before reaching hospital) and proportions given thrombolysis in hospital are 0.7, 0.7, and 0.6 in each ascending age group.

[†] Australian data.

Methodological concerns with the NNT and its population extensions

I have presented a simplified description of the value of the NNT and its population extensions. There are a number of methodological issues to point out, such as the fact that an event prevented does not include any value to that event—is it the same if it is in a person aged 25 or 85? This makes it difficult to apply in cost-effectiveness analyses.[12] I have said that the NNT is easily understood and applied by clinicians, and I have some evidence to back this up,[13] although others have found understanding by clinicians to be variable and not always correct.[14] Others have concerns of how the NNT relates to various subpopulations,[15] which we have tried to address in the next section.

Referring to your own population

It is also possible to refer these numbers to a population of relevance to you. To illustrate this, we can examine alternative secondary prevention strategies after heart attack (myocardial infarction or MI).

There are a couple more terms and formulae (see Appendix D at the end of this chapter for the calculations)!

Number to be treated in your population (NTP) 'the number of people *in your population* who will be eligible for the treatment' and number of events prevented in your population (NEPP) 'the number of events prevented by the intervention *in your population*'.

Let us return to our General Practice population of 10,000 people. The implementation of guidelines for the secondary prevention of MI will require 176 patients to be treated with aspirin, 147 patients with beta-blockers and with ACE-inhibitors and 157 patients with statins (NTP).[16] The benefit expressed as NEPP will range from 1.91 to 2.96 deaths prevented per year for aspirin and statins respectively. The drug cost per year varies from £1940 for aspirin to £60,525 for statins. Assuming incremental changes only (for those not already on treatment), aspirin post-MI will be added for 37 patients and produce 0.40 of a death prevented per year at a drug cost of £410 and statins will be added for 120 patients and prevent 2.26 deaths per year at a drug cost of £46,150. This costing includes only the drug costs, and not the additional costs of the medical encounter. It allows us to com-pare between the different drugs, as the non-drug costs should be

---

Box 4.1 **Example for Oldham**

In 2003, we examined prescribing patterns for patients who had had a myocardial infarction in General Practices in Oldham, Greater Manchester. The table shows the benefits from the treatment, and the potential to increase this if guidelines are to be followed.

	NEPP	NEPP*	NEPP Inc
Aspirin	20.23	22.13	1.9
B blockers	20.23	42.69	22.5
Statins	29.93	38.66	8.7

NEPP (number of events prevented, deaths and re-infarctions) = number of deaths prevented each year within the Oldham population aged 50+ according to current prescribing practices; NEPP* is the number of events prevented within this population if all practices prescribed each drug to 90% of post AMI as recommended in the National Service Framework for CHD; NEPP Inc is the incremental number of events prevented going from current practice to meet the National Service Framework targets.

similar between different drug regimes. As the cost of drugs change over time, for example with the movement of statins to generic prescription as patents expire, the differential costs between drug treatments should be reduced.

These measures, when related to the local population, could be used for health policy decision making in assigning priorities to alternative interventions. They can also be used for hospital populations.

Population decision analysis

Decision analysis is a technique, used by health economists, as a structured way of comparing the implications of alternative courses of action. In the clinical setting, we might examine a sequence of performing a diagnostic test, offering treatment or not based on the result, and examining the impact of this treatment on a particular health outcome. It has been suggested that this can be extended to the population setting, as a way of examining the population impact of an intervention.[17]

We have used decision analysis to estimate the population impact of alternative interventions for stroke, associated with increasing access to technology.[18]

We might note that roughly the same incremental impact is seen by adding the lowest technology option (aspirin for all) as the highest technology option (urgent CT scan and thrombolysis).

Table 4.6 Decision analysis to show impact on stroke population of low to high technology[18]

	Percentage who are dead or dependent 6-months after the stroke
No intervention	61.5%
Low technology (aspirin 2–4 weeks later)	61.0%
Intermediate technology (add organised stroke unit and anticoagulation if in atrial fibrillation)	58.3%
High technology (add CT scan and early aspirin)	57.9%
Very high technology (add urgent CT scan and thrombolysis if indicated)	57.5%

Health impact assessment, health needs assessment and summary measures of population health

There are a number of measures which either describe the impact on a population of a programme (which may or may not be designed to impact on health) or assess the health needs of a population. The similarity of terminology and overlap with the population impact measures just described requires some description here. I propose to offer a brief introduction to these measures with references to more extensive readings.

Health impact assessment

Health impact assessment (HIA) is the assessment of the potential health effects, positive or negative, of a particular project, programme, or policy on a population. It has been defined as 'a combination of procedures, methods and tools by which a policy, programme or project may be judged as to its potential effects on the health of a population, and the distribution of those effects within the population'.[19] The importance of this reflects the fact that a new project (such as the building of a new airport) may have unintended health consequences. Planners will have to show if there is any environmental impact of such a development, and if HIA is implemented, will also have to show the health impact on the population. The whole area is fully described in Kemm, Parry, and Palmer, 2004.[20] HIA is often considered as part of an environmental impact assessment (EIA), such as in the Canadian process which integrates health, social, and environmental aspects.[21] An impact assessment of the health effects of air pollution attributable to transport has been made for Manila (quoted in[22]). Based on a population of 9 million, the estimates included: 1300 deaths, 45 000 emergency room visits, 11 million 'restricted activity days', 35 million respiratory symptom days, and a cost of over 5 billion pesos. These results helped define public policy.

Health needs assessment

Health needs assessment (HNA) is the determination of the health needs of a particular community or population. There are five steps as described by the UK Health Development Agency (http://www. hda-online.org.uk/documents/hna.pdf.):

1 Getting started;

2 Identifying the health priorities for the population;

3 Assessing the specific health priority;

4 Planning and pulling it all together;

5 Evaluation.

HNA is a valuable tool. Its main benefit, I believe, is that those responsible for health planning have some kind of framework to use. The process would benefit from a more standardized method for making measures of health benefit at the population level, and it is this that our population impact measures may be able to provide.

Summary measures of population health

Murray and Lopez developed the concept of the 'global burden of disease'. They and colleagues identified a series of methods for measuring the burden of avoidable illness, which included both mortality and morbidity. They defined the term 'disability adjusted life year' (DALY) which extended the more traditional outcome measure of the 'quality adjusted life year' (QALY).[23,24] Health-adjusted life expectancy (HALE) adds a measure of quality of life to health expectancy,[25] and adjusts life expectancy for the amount of time spent in less than perfect health. An industry developed to teach health professionals how to make these measures of the burden of illness for their communities, and the measures are included in the World Health Report[26] where they have made an important impact.

Comparative risk assessment (CRA) is defined by WHO as 'the systematic evaluation of the changes in population health that result from modifying the population's exposure to a risk factor or a group of risk factors'.[22] While the mathematics can be daunting, the methodological issues require a depth of investigation and a number of interesting results are already available. For example, it is estimated that 39 per cent of the total disease burden, in the year 2000, resulted from the joint effects of 20 selected leading risk factors in 14 epidemiological subregions of the world.[27] The main problem with the measures has been their complexity and the level of understanding that is required by policy makers to translate the findings into health policy. The population impact measures which we have described attempt to produce both a more simple approach and one that can be related to a clear population base.

Key summary points

+ *The Student.* There are a number of ways of estimating the population impact of both risk factors and of interventions. The choice of measure should be determined by the availability of data and the use to which the result is to be put.

+ *The Practitioner.* Population impact measures are a new way of describing the population impact of risks or interventions, of relevance to a local population.

+ *The Policy-maker.* There are a number of methods of assessing the health gain of an intervention and the health impact of a risk factor. Health policy should incorporate health impacts on the population, and use locally relevant data for local decision-making.

Appendix A. Population Attributable Risk (PAR)

PAR is calculated as follows: For a dichotomous relative risk (such as being a cigarette smoker or not):

$$PAR = \frac{P_e(RR - 1)}{1 + P_e(RR - 1)}$$

For a series of relative risks (such as examining the risks associated with various levels or 'doses' of cigarette smoking):

$$Level\ i\ PAR = \frac{P_{ei}(RR_i - 1)}{1 + \sum_{i=1}^{k} Pe_i(RR_i - 1)}$$

$$Overall\ PAR = \frac{\sum_{i=1}^{k} P_{ei}(RR_i - 1)}{1 + \sum_{i=1}^{k} P_{ei}(RR_i - 1)}$$

where P_e is the proportion of the population exposed to the risk factor.

Appendix B. Population Impact Number of Eliminating a Risk factor (PIN-ER-*t*)

We saw above that the formula for the PAR is:

$$P_e(RR-1)/\ 1 + P_e(RR-1)$$

If we add to the formula I_p, the incidence of the disease outcome in the population, this will give the proportion of that incidence which is attributable to the exposure under examination. If we then add the number of people in the population, N, we will have the numbers of people in that population whose outcome is attributable to the exposure. All that is left to do is to add the time period over which the outcome is measured. The term is the Population Impact Number of Eliminating a Risk factor (PIN-ER-*t*), and is defined as 'the potential number of disease events prevented in your population over the next *t* years by eliminating a risk factor'. The full formula is $N{*}I_p{*}$ $[P_e(RR-1)/\ 1 + P_e(RR-1)]$.

Appendix C. Disease Impact Number (DIN) and Population Impact Number (PIN)

The Disease Impact Number (DIN) is calculated by 1/(absolute risk reduction × proportion of people with the disease who are exposed to the intervention). The Population Impact Number (PIN) is calculated by 1/(absolute risk reduction × proportion of people with the disease who are exposed to the intervention × proportion of the total population with the disease of interest).

Appendix D. Number to be Treated in your Population (NTP) and Number of Events Prevented in your Population (NEPP)

Number to be Treated in your Population (NTP) = Population size $*$ $P_e{*}\ P_d$ where P_e is the proportion of the diseased population eligible for treatment and P_d is the proportion of the population with the disease.

Number of Events Prevented in your Population (NEPP) = Population size $*$ P_e* P_d* Baseline risk $*$ RRR (This can also be expressed as: NTP $*$ Baseline risk $*$ RRR; or; NTP $*$ 1/NNT; or Population size/PIN).

References

1 Rothman K. J. and Greenland S. *Modern Epidemiology*. Philadelphia: Lippincott-Raven, 1998.

2 Levin M. L. The occurrence of lung cancer in man. *Acta Unio Inter Contra Cancrum* 1953; **19**: 531.

3 Heller R. F., Dobson A. J., Attia J., Page J. H. Impact numbers: measures of risk factor impact on the whole population from case control and cohort studies. *Journal of Epidemiology and Community Health* 2002; **56**: 606–10.

4 Doll R. and Peto R. Mortality in relation to smoking: 20 years' observations on male British doctors. *BMJ* 1976; **2**: 1525–36.

5 Heller R. F. and Dobson A. J. Disease impact number and population impact number: a population perspective to measures of risk and benefit. *BMJ* 2000; **321**: 950–2.

6 Heller R. F., Buchan I., Edwards R., Lyratzopoulos G., McElduff P., St Leger S. Communicating risks at the population level: application of population impact numbers. *BMJ* 2003; **327**: 1162–5.

7 McPherson K., Britton A., Causer L. *Coronary Heart Disease. Estimating the impact of changes in risk factors*. London: The Stationery Office: National Heart Forum, 2002.

8 Morgenstern H. and Bursic E. A method for using epidemiologic data to estimate the potential impact of an intervention on the health status of a target population. *Journal of Community Health* 1982; **7**: 292–309.

9 Browner W. S. Estimating the impact of risk factor modification programs. *Am. J. Epidemiol.* 1986; **123**: 143–53.

10 Laupacis A., Sackett D. L., Roberts R. S. An assessment of clinically useful measures of the consequences of treatment. *N. Engl. J. of Med.* 1988; **318**: 1728–33.

11 Heller R. F., Powell H., O'Connell R. L., D'Este K., Lim L. L. Trends in the hospital management of unstable angina. *Journal of Epidemiology and Community Health* 2001; **55**: 483–6.

12 Kristiansen I. S. and Gyrd-Hansen D. Cost-effectiveness analysis based on the number-needed-to-treat: common sense or non-sense? *Health Econ.* 2004; **13**: 9–19.

13 Heller R. F., Sandars J., Patterson L., McElduff P. GPs' and physicians' interpretation of risks, benefits and diagnosis test results. *Fam. Pract.* 2004; **21**: 155–9.

14 Kristiansen I. S., Gyrd-Hansen D., Nexoe J., Nielsen J. B. Number needed to treat: easily understood and intutitively meaningful? Theoretical considerations and a randomised trial. *Journal of Clinical Epidemiology* 2002; **55**: 888–92.

15 Wu L. A. and Kottke T. E. Number needed to treat: caveat emptor. *J. Clin. Epidemiol.* 2001; **54**: 111–16.

16 Heller R. F., Edwards R., McElduff P. Implementing guidelines in primary care: can population impact measures help? *BMC Public Health* 2003; **3**: 7.

17 Hersh A. L., Black W. C., Tosteson A. N. Estimating the population impact of an intervention: a decision-analytic approach. *Stat. Methods Med. Res.* 1999; **8**: 311–30.

18 Heller R. F., Langhorne P., James E. Improving stroke outcome: the benefits of increasing availability of technology. *Bulletin of the World Health Organization* 2000; **78**: 1337–43.

19 European Centre for Health Policy. Gothenburg Consensus Paper. 1999. WHO Regional Office for Europe.

20 Kemm J., Parry J., Palmer S. *Health Impact Assessment—Concepts, theory, techniques and applications.* Oxford: Oxford University Press, 2004.

21 Kwiatkowski R. E. and Ooi M. Integrated environmental impact assessment: a Canadian example. *Bull. World Health Organ* 2003; **81**: 434–8.

22 Kjellstrom T., van Kerkhoff L., Bammer G., McMichael T. Comparative assessment of transport risks–how it can contribute to health impact assessment of transport policies. *Bull. World Health Organ* 2003; **81**: 451–7.

23 Murray C. J. L. and Lopez A. D. *The Global Burden of Disease: a comprehensive assessment of mortality and disability from diseases, injuries and risk factors in 1990 and projected to 2020.* Cambridge, MA: Harvard School of Public Health on behalf of the World Health Organization and The World Bank, 1966.

24 Mathers C. D., Stein C., Ma Fat D., Rao C., Inoue M., Tomijima N., Berbard C., Lopez A. D., and Murray C. J. L. *Global Burden of Disease 2000: version 2 methods and results.* Geneva: World Health Organization, Global Programme on Evidence for Health Policy Discussion Paper No. 50, 2002. Internet communication at web site http://www.who.int/evidence/bod.

25 Manuel D. and Schultz S. Using linked data to calculate summary measures of population health: Health-adjusted life expectancy of people with Diabetes Mellitus. *Population Health Metrics* 2004; **2**: 4.

26 World Health Organization. *The World Health Report 2002: reducing risks, promoting healthy life.* Geneva: World Health Organization, 2002.

27 Ezzati M., Hoorn S. V., Rodgers A., Lopez A. D., Mathers C. D., Murray C. J. Estimates of global and regional potential health gains from reducing multiple major risk factors. *Lancet* 2003; **362**: 271–80.

28 Attia J., Page J., Heller, R. F., Dobson A. J. Impact numbers in health policy decisions. *Journal of Epidemiology and Community Health* 2002; **56**: 600–5.

Chapter 5

Evaluating population-based risks and interventions

This chapter discusses the appropriateness of 'levels of evidence' which place systematic reviews of randomized controlled trials as the highest level of evidence, and proposes a new 'population evidence hierarchy'.

In the previous chapter, we have seen that accurate estimates of relative risk and relative risk reduction are essential to determine the population impact of risks and interventions. These estimates come from research studies and the synthesis of as many studies as possible. Before going much further, we need to assess the quality of these studies, and a number of attempts have been made to put study quality into a 'hierarchy of evidence'. Much of this work has related to clinically relevant research evidence, and this chapter starts by attempting to define the levels of evidence of relevance to population research.

The hierarchy of evidence has been used in evidence-based medicine to encourage the use of evidence that has been derived using the highest quality of research design. This has built on the initial categorization of research designs adapted from the Canadian Taskforce on Periodic Health Examination[1] by the US Preventive Services Taskforce. The US Taskforce was convened by the US Public Health Service to 'rigorously evaluate clinical research in order to assess the merits of preventive measures, including screening tests, counselling, immunizations, and chemoprophylaxis'.[2]

This places the randomized controlled trial (RCT) at the top of the hierarchy, although others have inserted systematic reviews above the RCT. The US Preventive Services Taskforce is developing its third report at the time of writing this, and has added the quality of the study design (internal validity) to the type of study in making its assessment. There is also a recognition that the external validity of the study—can you generalize the results to your own population of interest?—is relevant to a decision about the value of a research study. Even well-designed and well-conducted studies may not supply the evidence needed if the studies examine a highly selected population of little relevance to yours.

Hierarchy of research design as of 1990[2]

I: Evidence obtained from at least one properly randomized controlled trial.

II-1: Evidence obtained from well-designed controlled trials without randomization.

II-2: Evidence obtained from well-designed cohort or case-control analytic studies, preferably from more than one centre or research group.

II-3: Evidence obtained from multiple time series with or without the intervention. Dramatic results in uncontrolled experiments (such as the results of the introduction of penicillin treatment in the 1940s) could also be regarded as this type of evidence.

III: Opinions of respected authorities, based on clinical experience, descriptive studies and case reports, or reports of expert committees.

Hierarchy of evidence as of 2003[3]

- ◆ Systematic reviews and meta-analyses
- ◆ RCTs with definitive results
- ◆ RCTs with non-definitive results
- ◆ Cohort studies
- ◆ Case-control studies
- ◆ Cross-sectional surveys
- ◆ Case reports.

The currently accepted hierarchy of evidence is relevant for clinical practice, particularly in relation to the use of pharmaceutical agents, where the RCT is clearly the most relevant, and essential, study design. However, much public health research is not suitable for the RCT, and even in areas where the RCT might be possible, they are few and far between. Thus, much public health decision-making needs to rely on types of evidence that do not figure at the top of the hierarchy of evidence. Suggestions have been made to develop alternative hierarchies, or to replace the hierarchy with a typology or framework which emphasizes the appropriateness of the methodology to the question being asked. This is important, because a poorly performed RCT, or one on a non-representative or non-relevant population, may produce less useful evidence than a study 'lower' on the research hierarchy.

Petticrew and Roberts[3] have adapted a framework from Muir Gray, and suggest that we first identify the research question being asked, and then identify the most appropriate research design to answer this question before we assign a hierarchy to the evidence produced. As Habicht and colleagues argue,[4] the main objective of an evaluation is to influence decisions. The nature and complexity of the evaluation should depend on the decision to be made once the evaluation has been performed. They provide two axes along which an evaluation might be performed 'What do you want to measure?' and 'How sure do you want to be?' Table 5.1 shows how this might relate to programmes designed to control diarrhoeal diseases.

I think it would be helpful to expand on the types of study that can provide good evidence for public health decision-making, and offer a classification here. This assumes that the standard appraisal of each study has assured acceptable quality. As Rychetnik and colleagues have pointed out in a profound paper on this subject,[5] the study design is not enough to decide on whether the results of a study are adequate markers of quality to be of use in public health decision-making. They define credibility, completeness and transferability as being of importance beyond the study design itself. I have adopted their classification in my own schema in Table 5.2.

While the traditional quality assessments go in ascending order in this table, the criteria of completeness and transferability tend to go in descending order. This raises the challenge of designing studies that capture real-life exposures rather than the artificiality of a research study—to which we will return later in Chapter 7

Table 5.1 Examples of types of evaluations of diarrhoeal diseases control programmes[4]

How sure do you want to be?	What do you want to measure?			
	Provision	Utilization	Coverage	Impact
Adequacy	Changes in availability of oral rehydration therapy (ORT) in health centres	Changes in numbers of ORT packages distributed in health centres	Measurement of percentage of diarrhoeal episodes treated with ORT in the population	Measurement of trends in diarrhoeal mortality in intervention area
Plausibility	As above, but comparing with control services	As above, but comparing with control services	Comparison of ORT coverage between intervention and control areas (or dose–response)	Comparison of diarrhoeal mortality trends between intervention and control areas (or dose–response)
Probability	As above, but intervention and control services would have been randomized	As above, but intervention and control services would have been randomized	As above, with previous randomization	As above, with previous randomization

Table 5.2 The population evidence hierarchy

Direction of external validity (for generalising the results to your population) →

Study type*	Requirement for use in public health decision-making		
	Credibility	Completeness	Transferability
Randomized controlled trials (or systematic reviews of trials) with individuals as the unit of randomization	If performed on representative and relevant population with appropriate exposure/intervention	If outcomes cover the interests of the stakeholders; include intended and unintended outcomes; the efficiency of the outcome (such as cost-effectiveness)	If there is information on the detail of the intervention (including its stage of development), the context in which it is introduced and any interaction between intervention and context
Cluster randomized controlled trial (or systematic reviews of trials)	As above, and if cluster design (and the sample size implication) is included in analysis		
Quasi-experimental design	If appropriate comparison groups are included, baseline comparability and dose-response relationship between acceptance of intervention, risk factor change of intervention, and outcome are demonstrated[6]	If negative results appropriately interpreted	
Cohort studies and high quality clinical databases	If propensity for exposure to risk factor or intervention examined		
Before/after studies (time series)	If compared with other time period or population without the intervention		
Case control studies	If exposures and population representative of your population of interest		
Ecologic studies	If supported by individual level data		

← Direction of internal validity (for avoiding bias)

* Qualitative studies which may contribute to population evidence are not considered here.

on surveillance using e-science. We will also return to the use of evidence in policy-making later (Chapter 10), where we will see that the burden of illness is another factor, beyond the quality of the evidence for an intervention, which determines the introduction of a new policy.

You may also want to read other discussions of levels of evidence, such as that produced by the Oxford Centre for Evidence-Based Medicine, although most of these relate to clinical rather than population decision-making (see http://www.cebm.net/levels_of_evidence.asp). Of relevance is the importance of ensuring that non-randomized studies are well designed, and the TREND statement has been developed to improve the reporting quality of such studies.[7]

Evaluating community interventions

Currently in the UK there is a drive to reduce inequalities through the development of neighbourhood initiatives. These have a focus beyond health, and in the current set of programmes, health has taken a back seat to initiatives to reduce crime, increase educational and housing opportunities and reduce unemployment (although these other measures would be expected to have a health impact). They have their recent historical roots in the Healthy Cities programme adopted and sponsored by WHO. The programmes can be described under the term 'regeneration and neighbourhood change' and include many area-based initiatives, new deal for communities and follow the development of 'action zones' which have included Health Action Zones.

These are mostly examples of decision-making in the absence of evidence. Most of these initiatives are just good ideas rather than reflecting the policy application of an evidence base. Worse than the lack of evidence supporting their introduction, they are frequently not (or poorly) evaluated. Baseline data to allow future evaluation are often not collected and if objectives are not clearly specified appropriate measures of outcome are difficult to make. The inclusion of a control or comparison group is unusual, and the development of the initiative in the context of a well-designed experiment is rare. Many of the 'evaluations' of politically inspired programmes are nothing more than lists of what is being done, or of process—has the community come together to work on the scheme, has the money been spent, have new roads/jobs/green spaces been developed? There is usually a disparity between the timeframes necessary for achieving or demonstrating change and the political necessity of demonstrating progress. The politicization of health initiatives has been described as often counter-scientific.[8]

Community-based intervention trials

While most randomized controlled trials randomize the individual patient, public health interventions are frequently more appropriately evaluated by randomizing the population or community. Some such trials involve more complex interventions than the typical individual patient intervention, and hence have a special set of problems. One of the best described community intervention trials is the COMMIT study, where a number of pairs of communities were randomly allocated to intervention or control.[9] There are a number of methodological implications of complex and community-based interventions (see the Medical Research Council web site: http://www.mrc.ac.uk/pdf-mrc_cpr.pdf). Kirkwood and colleagues have drawn on experience of research in developing countries to suggest design issues of relevance to community-based interventions.[6] They make the point that in this type of evaluation, even when a randomized controlled trial is used, the unit of randomization is a community or cluster of individuals rather than an individual. This requires a special set of methodological markers of quality. Often, even the cluster randomized trial is not suitable, in which case other design qualities should be borne in mind when deciding whether an outcome can truly be attributed to the intervention. In a quasi-experimental study, randomization is not performed, but some kind of comparison group is included to the population offered the intervention, preferably with before–after comparisons also included in both groups. When considering other study designs, such as the quasi-experimental, Kirkwood and colleagues suggest several features that permit an observed change to be attributed to the intervention. These are shown in Box 5.1.

> ## Box 5.1 Suggestions that observed change can be attributed to the intervention
>
> - Existence of a sensible hypothesis
> - Baseline comparability between groups
> - Risk factor has changed more in intervention than comparison group
> - Outcome factor has changed more in intervention than comparison group
> - Dose-response relationship between acceptance of intervention, risk factor change and outcome.
>
> From Kirkwood et al.[6]

What can we do when we can't do a trial—is observation enough?

There has been considerable discussion about the relative merits of trials and observational studies. In some circumstances observational studies may be the only practicable option.[10] Where investigators require longer follow-up periods, data on a wide range of possible heath outcomes, and timely evidence from representative settings in rapidly changing policy and health care environments, observational studies may be the preferred option. For evaluating the effects of behavioural and lifestyle modification, Stampfer has said that observation is the preferred means, and lists a number of problems with reliance on the RCT.[11] Britton and colleagues examined differences between randomized and non-randomized studies and concluded[12] that:

- A well-designed non-randomized study is preferable to a small, poorly designed and exclusive RCT.
- RCTs should be pragmatic by including as wide a range of practice settings as possible. Study populations should be representative of all patients currently being treated for the condition.
- Exclusions for administrative convenience should be rejected.

There is a body of evidence that observational data usually come to the same conclusion as RCTs. Concato[13] and Benson[14] and their colleagues reviewed a number of different studies of the same topic, and found considerable concordance between the results of trials and observational studies. Concato searched Medline for papers in five medical journals between 1991 and 1995 for meta-analyses of RCTs and either cohort or case-control studies that assessed the same intervention. For five topics and 99 reports there were similar results from RCT and observational studies. The authors concluded that well-designed observational studies do not overestimate treatment effects, that observational results are less heterogeneous than RCTs, and more likely to include a broad representation of the population at risk. Benson searched Index Medicus and Cochrane 1985–1998 to find observational studies that compared two or more treatments or interventions for the same condition. For each treatment, observational study results were combined and then compared with RCT results. There were 136 reports of 19 treatments, and the results were similar (except 2 of 19 analyses observed a treatment effect outside the 95 per cent CI of the RCTs). The authors concluded that there is a need to exploit clinically-rich databases to see how they can be used (and avoid the usual criticism that observational studies are distorted by unrecognized confounders).

A furious correspondence followed in the journal, mainly from RCT supporters. In response, Concato *et al.* said[13]:

> We sympathize with all who find intellectual security in randomization as a method of ensuring the validity of study results. Surely, however, other methods (matching, stratification, adjustment and restriction) are available to ensure validity when randomization is absent.

After the above papers were written, a major controversy has arisen in relation to the effects of postmenopausal hormone replacement therapy (HRT) and cardiovascular disease. For years, observational studies had shown that women who take postmenopausal oestrogens are less likely to develop heart disease. RCTs have, however, shown an excess of cardiovascular disease among those randomly allocated to oestrogen therapy. This finding has cast doubt on the conclusions discussed above, although the last word has not been said on the issue.[15] The figure we reproduce from the review shows how for all outcome

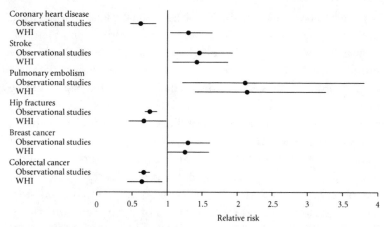

Fig. 5.1 Relation between postmenopausal HT and various clinical end points in observational studies and in the Women's Health Initiative (WHI).[15]

measures other than coronary heart disease, observational studies and trials provided similar estimates of effect.

A similar problem has arisen with the results of observational studies on antioxidant vitamins, which have shown inverse relationships with cardiovascular disease not confirmed by RCTs.[16–18] The suggestion has been made that the vitamin differences were due to their being proxy indicators of factors that protect against the disease outcomes, and that careful examination of potential confounders along the lifecourse, should help avoid erroneous results from observational studies.[17] The point about a need to explore and understand confounders more thoroughly has been made by Concato and Horwitz,[16] and Vandenbroucke suggests that observational studies should be performed according to a set of restrictions (by research topic, design and analysis) to enhance their value.[18]

Much of this debate has reflected on clinical interventions, and Victora and colleagues have written persuasively about the need to expand the thinking on the distinction between the RCT and observational studies where public health interventions are concerned.[19] Due to the complexity of the causal chain between the intervention and the outcome in many non-clinical interventions, there are many opportunities for effect modification in different populations—for example there are at last six steps between an intervention of health worker training in nutrition counselling leading to the improved outcome of increased weight gain in a developing country. They make the point that to interpret the results of a RCT in such a situation, it is essential to supplement the results with observational studies on the intermediate steps of the causal chain (such as whether the messages were actually transmitted to mothers) if we are to interpret the results of such a trial correctly. Victora and colleagues have suggested a taxonomy of design—probability (RCT), plausibility (non-random observational comparisons involving a comparison group) and adequacy (observation of trends) which may be useful.[19,4]

Whatever the merits of observational studies versus trials, there are few population-based trials, and observation will have to be the mainstay of the evidence used for decision-making. Use of the population evidence hierarchy might help the population policy-maker decide how to use various levels of evidence.

Key summary points

- *The Student.* While the randomized controlled trial (and systematic reviews of numbers of trials) provide the most internally valid evidence, these are often not feasible for examining population-level risks and interventions and suffer from lack of external validity (cannot be applied in a real-life setting to your population).

- *The Practitioner.* A new hierarchy of evidence for application at the population level is suggested, which encourages the use of alternative study designs based on their credibility, completeness, transferability and hence usefulness.

- *The Policy-maker.* It is important not to deny the use of evidence for policy-making just because it has not come from a systematic review of RCTs.

References

1 The periodic health examination. Canadian Task Force on the Periodic Health Examination. *Can. Med. Assoc. J.* 1979; **121**: 1193–254.

2 Lawrence R. S., Mickalide A. D., Kamerow D. B., Woolf S. H. Report of the US Preventive Services Task Force. *JAMA* 1990; **263**: 436–7.

3 Petticrew M. and Roberts H. Evidence, hierarchies, and typologies: horses for courses. *J. Epidemiol. Community Health* 2003; **57**: 527–9.

4 Habicht J. P., Victora C. G., Vaughan J. P. Evaluation designs for adequacy, plausibility and probability of public health programme performance and impact. *Int. J. Epidemiol.* 1999; **28**: 10–8.

5 Rychetnik L., Frommer M., Hawe P., Shiell A. Criteria for evaluating evidence on public health interventions. *J. Epidemiol. Community Health* 2002; **56**: 119–27.

6 Kirkwood B. R., Cousens S. N., Victora C. G., de Z, I. Issues in the design and interpretation of studies to evaluate the impact of community-based interventions. *Trop. Med. Int. Health* 1997; **2**: 1022–9.

7 Des J., Lyles C., Crepaz N. Improving the reporting quality of nonrandomized evaluations of behavioral and public health interventions: the TREND statement. *Am. J. Public Health* 2004; **94**: 361–6.

8 Rosenstock L. and Lee L. J. Attacks on science: the risks to evidence-based policy. *Am. J. Public Health* 2002; **92**: 14–8.

9 Thompson B., Lichtenstein E., Corbett K., Nettekoven L., Feng Z. Durability of tobacco control efforts in the 22 Community Intervention Trial for Smoking Cessation (COMMIT) communities two years after the end of intervention. *Health Educ. Res.* 2000; **15**: 353–66.

10 Black N. Why we need observational studies to evaluate the effectiveness of health care. *BMJ* 1996; **312**: 1215–18.

11 Stampfer M. Observational epidemiology is the preferred means of evaluating effects of behavioral and lifestyle modification. *Control Clin. Trials* 1997; **18**: 494–9.

12 Britton A., McKee M., Black N., McPherson K., Sanderson C., Bain C. Choosing between randomised and non-randomised studies: a systematic review. *Health Technol. Assess.* 1998; **2**: 1–124.

13 Concato J., Shah N., Horwitz R. I. Randomized, controlled trials, observational studies, and the hierarchy of research designs. *N. Engl. J. Med.* 2000; **342**: 1887–92.

14 Benson K. and Hartz A. J. A comparison of observational studies and randomized, controlled trials. *N. Engl. J. Med.* 2000; **342**: 1878–86.

15 Michels K. B. and Manson J. E. Postmenopausal hormone therapy: a reversal of fortune. *Circulation* 2003; **107**: 1830–3.

16 Concato J. and Horwitz R. I. Beyond randomised versus observational studies. *Lancet* 2004; **363**: 1660–1.

17 Lawlor D. A., Davey S. G., Kundu D., Bruckdorfer K. R., Ebrahim S. Those confounded vitamins: what can we learn from the differences between observational versus randomised trial evidence? *Lancet* 2004; **363**: 1724–7.

18 Vandenbroucke J. P. When are observational studies as credible as randomised trials? *Lancet* 2004; **363**: 1728–31.

19 Victora C. G., Habicht J. P., Bryce J. Evidence-based public health: moving beyond randomized trials. *Am. J. Public Health* 2004; **94**: 400–5.

Chapter 6

Getting the outcome measure right

This chapter considers the individual and the population approaches to assessing health outcomes. Death, hospitalization, quality of life, cost, disability, inequality and health literacy are considered and compared as possible outcome measures.

Epidemiology concerns 'exposures' and 'outcomes', and epidemiologic explorations aim to discover associations between the two. If we are going to use and implement the results of such explorations, we will have to ensure that the outcomes identified are those which can be related to a policy decision. There is a tendency in much health policy-making to focus on process measures, rather than on the actual outcomes of policy on health status. In addition to making a plea to examine outcome rather than process, I also want to ensure that we measure outcomes that are appropriate to the policy issue.

The use of outcome data will depend critically on the questions that lay behind their collection in the first place. Why were the data colleted? Are they going to be used for individual patient care decisions, or for public health policy-making? Are they attempting to reflect the impact of a health system, of a particular intervention aimed at individuals or communities, or of a risk behaviour? Is it an evaluation of efficacy—how well can an intervention work in the best circumstances—or effectiveness—how well can an intervention work in real life? What is going to be done, and by whom, with the results of the outcome data?

Consistent with our overall theme of the individual and the population, let's first identify whether the use is for individuals or populations.

Health outcomes among individuals

Preventing death (living longer), preventing illness or disability, preventing use of health services such as hospitalization and improving quality of life are all outcomes which an individual might welcome. The UK Clearing House for Health Outcomes has offered a classification of health outcomes, by listing the instruments that can be used for their measurement. http://www.leeds.ac.uk/nuffield/infoservices/UKCH/about.html

Measures of health outcomes

+ Mortality
+ Complications/service morbidity
+ Disease-specific measures
+ Topic-specific measures (aspects of health)
+ Health-related behaviour
+ Multidimensional health status profiles
+ Multidimensional health status indices
+ Measures of service use
+ Reported symptoms and conditions.

While there are numerous methodological issues to discuss in relation to the measurement of such outcomes, I've picked out a few key points.

Mortality

This can be expressed as lives saved, deaths prevented or postponed and a relevant time factor is essential. It can be expressed in relative or absolute reduction terms, and can involve examination of event-free periods at different ages. The notion that we can save lives is also rather naive—we all have to die from something. Tan and Murphy have argued clearly that extending lives is a more appropriate measure to use and that trial results expressed in these terms may give a different impression than a reduction in mortality.[1]

Morbidity

This can be self-assessed or measured by use of health services. Morbidity can be a biased measure because health services may actually be a determinant of health rather than an outcome. Access to health services may be inequitable and thus a poor marker of health outcomes if used to assess differences in health across an inequality spectrum.

Perceived state of health or Quality of Life (QoL)

There are a number of ways of measuring QoL. An important outcome of any clinical intervention is the change in the subject's own perceived state of health. This can be categorized as health-related quality of life (HRQL), utility (preference-based health state), and daily life performance.[2] Measures can be a self-rated health assessment, or formal measures of QoL. These are either general measures which can provide a health profile (such as the [Short Form] SF-36 measure), or they can provide utility estimates to feed directly into cost-effectiveness or cost-utility analyses. Alternatively, a number of disease specific measures have been developed, such as those for heart disease, chronic lung disease or diabetes.

Health outcomes among groups

One way of going from the individual to the group is to aggregate the individual measures for group purposes. When we do this, we may use measures of health outcome that are relevant to the population. Thus, for example, we may use population impact measures for population decisions, rather than the number needed to treat for decisions involving individuals (see Chapter 4). It may be more appropriate to think in terms of avoidable mortality, as this will give us some clues about preventing it (see below). Among the special measures required for population-level decisions, however, are some of the following.

Health literacy

Nutbeam has defined health literacy as an important outcome, as it may be key to health promotion.[3,4] Health literacy may follow health promotion actions and may in turn be followed by intermediate health outcomes (modifiable determinants of health) which themselves lead to health and social outcomes such as mortality and morbidity. Health literacy can be classified as:

◆ *Basic/functional literacy*—sufficient basic skills in reading and writing to be able to function effectively in everyday situations, broadly compatible with the narrow definition of 'health literacy' referred to above.

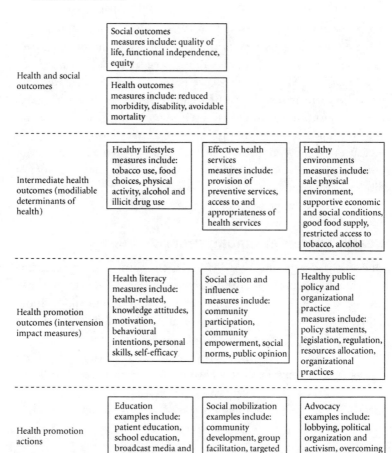

Fig. 6.1 Various levels of outcome from health promotion.[3]

♦ *Communicative/interactive* literacy—more advanced cognitive and literacy skills which, together with social skills, can be used to actively participate in everyday activities, to extract information and derive meaning from different forms of communication, and to apply new information to changing circumstances.

♦ *Critical literacy*—more advanced cognitive skills which, together with social skills, can be applied to critically analyse information, and to use this information to exert greater control over life events and situations.

Figure 6.1 shows how health literacy fits in the hierarchy of exposures and outcomes of health promotion.

Health economics

A full discussion of health economics is beyond the scope of this book, but it must be mentioned in a section on population health outcomes because of the importance and relevance to population health policy-making.

Cost-effectiveness, cost-utility and cost–benefit analyses (CEA, CUA and CBA) provide methods for comparing relative costs and health gains of different interventions—a common outcome measure is produced to allow such comparison. The quality-adjusted life year (QALY) is the most commonly used of these measures in CEA or CUA: it allows adjustment for quality of life as well as mortality, adjustment for length of benefit, and can be adjusted for societal views on equity.[5] While this might be suitable for government level spending decisions, and is used for example by the UK National Institute of Clinical Excellence (NICE), different types of analysis may be suitable for different levels of decision-making, hence this might not be suitable at a more local level.

These measures have a number of potential advantages, the main one being that they provide a method for comparing relative costs and health gains of different interventions—a common outcome measure is produced to allow such comparison. Despite this, they are not often used in practice. There have been a number of criticisms, the main ones being the difficulty of providing context-specific relevance and the inherent biases in the measurement of eliciting values (utilities) associated with particular outcomes. The use of life expectancy in the calculation does add an indication of the length of time over which a benefit might be gained, but ignores the value of a benefit at specific ages as well as the incorporation of the disease duration and the differentiation of benefit associated with different durations. The measures are also difficult to use to assess the impact of interventions on health inequalities—they suffer from the lack of a population perspective: mostly the population values are obtained by summing values for individuals. The two main measures used are the DALY and the QALY.

The DALY (disability-adjusted life year) was developed to assess the burden of illness in a large population (such as a country). It combines disability (YLD—years of life lived with a disability, calculated from disease prevalence, disease duration and a disability severity weight) and mortality (years of life lost—YLL). It should be discounted (for future health effects being less important than current ones), and maybe should have age-weights (so that illness or death at different ages are given different weights).

QALY (quality adjusted life years). Here each life year is weighted by a value between 0 and 1 reflecting quality of life, where 0 is the worst case, usually death, and 1 is full health. Methods for deriving weights include standard gamble, time trade-off and the visual analogue scale. The derivation of these weights has been severely criticized,[6] the methods may not be repeatable and may be context-specific.

These are the outcomes used for CEA and CUA, although some restrict cost-effectiveness analysis to where the outcome is not given a value, just a quantity, such as potential years of life lost (PYYL). CBA uses the monetary value of the benefits rather than a measure of well-being as the outcome. Cost-consequence analysis evaluates inter-ventions by comparing the costs of different interventions against simpler, common, outcome measures.

We have discussed some of the attributes and uses of population burden of illness measures, such as the DALY, in Chapter 4.

Health inequality as an outcome

There are major geographic between-population disparities in patterns of health. Within national populations, we have been aware of health inequalities for a long time. Many diseases are more likely to occur among those who are at the lower than the higher end of any social or income scale, at least in part due to differences in risk-taking behaviour. There is also variation in the quality of health care provided for those who are at the more deprived end of the social spectrum, and this may be due both to problems of the delivery of care and of patient expectations. The whole topic is huge and complex, but at least some thought needs to be given to what outcome measure is used when we discuss health inequalities. I'd also like to restrict the discussion to the outcome measure: it is a different issue to consider the 'exposure' measure for inequality as well.

Much political capital has been made of the widening gap between those at the extremes of the social spectrum. In the UK, this has driven much of the public health agenda in the National Health Service at the end of the twentieth and beginning of the twenty-first centuries. While there is little debate that those at the lowest end of the social spectrum have worse health outcomes than those at the top, however expressed, there is debate about whether the gap between them is widening or not. Much of this comes back to the debate about relative and absolute risk!

As Oliver has shown,[7,8] when the mortality gap in the UK is studied over time, the gap between the top and bottom social classes has widened only in relative terms: in absolute terms it had narrowed. This is also shown by the Australian New South Wales Chief Health Officer, who has taken the added step of examining health inequalities in mortality for those conditions where mortality might be potentially avoidable.[9] The approach to focus on potentially avoidable mortality uses methods developed by Tobias and colleagues in New Zealand,[10,11] and has been echoed by Nolte and McKee who find that the ranking of national health systems by mortality amenable to health care differs from ranking based on DALYs.[12]

Changes in population demographic characteristics can also influence the changing mortality gap between social extremes. Regidor[13] has shown that the variation in mortality inequalities between shrinking and growing areas can be attributable more to distribution bias than to health characteristics, and we have shown that a proportion of the reduction in mortality between 1970–72 and 1991–93 was due to upward mobility and a changing social class distribution.[14]

Whether we express the gap in relative or absolute terms is a matter of debate, and depends on the underlying philosophic approach. Are we more interested in some measure of inequality, or in the health status of the population as a whole, or whether the health of the most disadvantaged group is improving or not? This has been discussed in Chapter 3 in relation to the Rawls' minimax principle.

Critical appraisal

Whatever the outcome measure used, it is important to be clear about the quality, and the 'users guides' to critical appraisal suggest a number of criteria by which outcome measures should be assessed[15]—I have modified them here.

1 Does the outcome relate clearly to the question being asked in the study or to the study hypothesis?

2 Are appropriate outcomes assessed? Is a population perspective provided for the outcome measures?

3 Is there measurement error which could cause bias in the results?

4 Were there appropriate comparison groups?

5 Were there potential confounders that could have influenced the between-group comparisons?

6 Are the outcomes presented in a way that will help in policy decision-making?

Key summary points

- *The Student.* It is more important to assess health outcomes than the process of care, which may change but not lead to an improvement in health.

- *The Practitioner.* There are a number of population-based measures of health outcome which should be considered, beyond measures of individual outcome. A scheme for the critical appraisal of health outcomes should be followed in assessing their value.

♦ *The Policy-maker.* The choice of the appropriate health outcome to examine should be made in relation to the reason for the policy to be introduced in the first place. Please focus on outcome rather than process!

References

1 Tan L. B. and Murphy R. Shifts in mortality curves: saving or extending lives? *Lancet* 1999; **354**: 1378–81.

2 Stahl E., Jansson S. A., Jonsson A. C., Svensson K., Lundback B., Andersson F. Health-related quality of life, utility, and productivity outcomes instruments: ease of completion by subjects with COPD. *Health Qual. Life Outcomes* 2003; **1**: 18.

3 Nutbeam D. Health literacy as a public health goal: a challenge for contemporary health education and communication strategies into the 21st century. *Health Promot. Int.* 2000; **15**: 259–67.

4 Renkert S. and Nutbeam D. Opportunities to improve maternal health literacy through antenatal education: an exploratory study. *Health Promot. Int.* 2001; **16**: 381–8.

5 Williams A. QALYS and ethics: a health economist's perspective. *Soc. Sci. Med.* 1996; **43**: 1795–804.

6 Oliver A. Putting the quality into quality-adjusted life years. *J. Public Health Med.* 2003; **25**: 8–12.

7 Oliver A., Healey A., Le Grand J. Addressing health inequalities. *Lancet* 2002; **360**: 565–7.

8 Oliver A. On health inequality. *J. Public Health Med.* 2000; **22**: 454–6.

9 NSW Chief Health Officer. *Report of the NSW Chief Health Officer.* New South Wales, Australia, NSW Health, 2002.

10 Tobias M. and Jackson G. Avoidable mortality in New Zealand, 1981–97. *Aust. N. Z. J. Public Health* 2001; **25**: 12–20.

11 Tobias M. I. and Cheung J. Monitoring health inequalities: life expectancy and small area deprivation in New Zealand. *Popul. Health Metr.* 2003; **1**: 2.

12 Nolte E. and McKee M. Measuring the health of nations: analysis of mortality amenable to health care. *BMJ* 2003; **327**: 1129.

13 Regidor E., Calle M. E., Dominguez V., Navarro P. Inequalities in mortality in shrinking and growing areas. *J.Epidemiol. Community Health* 2002; **56**: 919–21.

14 Heller R. F., McElduff P., Edwards R. Impact of upward social mobility on population mortality: analysis with routine data. *BMJ* 2002; **325**: 134–6.

15 Naylor C. D. and Guyatt G. H. Users' guides to the medical literature. X. How to use an article reporting variations in the outcomes of health services. The Evidence-Based Medicine Working Group. *JAMA* 1996; **275**: 554–8.

Chapter 7

Public health informatics: the role of e-science in building the evidence base

This chapter identifies the importance of the revolution in information technology, which is transforming our ability to collect data of importance in building an evidence base for population health.

In Chapter 5, we discussed how one of the problems of producing the evidence base is that randomized controlled trials, traditionally thought to produce the best evidence, may have limitations for public health. There are many public health interventions which are introduced, for which evaluation opportunities are missed: there are many opportunities to explore causation which are being missed. The revolution in information technology has provided many of these opportunities, and this chapter aims to explore their scope.

Public Health Informatics is defined in an excellent (for the time) NIH Bibliography (http://www.nlm.nih.gov/pubs/cbm/phi2001.html), as

> The systematic application of information and computer sciences to public health practice, research, and learning. It is the discipline that integrates public health with information technology. The development of this field and dissemination of informatics knowledge and expertise to public health professionals is the key to unlocking the potential of information systems to improve the health of the nation.

A more operational definition is provided by Iain Buchan, my colleague in the Evidence for Population Health Unit in the University of Manchester, as: 'Knowledge, skills and tools for systematically creating information and managing knowledge to understand, protect and improve health in society.'

The need for public health informatics has been identified by the Centers for Disease Control (CDC) who have introduced a Fellowship programme saying that: 'Modern public health practice requires the increased development and use of sophisticated electronic systems to facilitate communication and data exchange among public health personnel at the local, state, and federal levels' (http://www.cdc.gov/ epo/dphsi/phifp/about.htm). The most obvious example of where the use of informatics is relevant to public health is in communicable disease control, where the tracking of the emergence of epidemics can be facilitated by computerized surveillance systems. CDC have extended this concept to bioterrorism detection. In less fraught times, information has long been known to be central to public health, and in the UK, information officers were part of the public health team in health authorities for years. The UK Public Health Observatory system has been established to produce data of relevance for public health and access to each regional observatory can easily be obtained through a central web site to allow for ease and speed of access to data (http://www.pho.org.uk/). Health informatics can be relevant to most public health functions, and as information technology develops over the twenty-first century, the field is likely to grow considerably.

Use of clinical data

It is possible to use data originally collected for clinical purposes to answer questions of public health relevance.[1]

Here are two examples of how collecting clinical data in population terms might be useful. The first uses population health methods to collect data on breast cancer survival and produce an online estimation of prognosis for use by individual patients and clinicians.[2] Figure 7.1 gives an example. While we can see how the clinician may use such data to offer prognosis to an individual patient, it is important to keep the database fresh to reflect recent advances in treatment which may change (we hope improve) the natural history of the condition.

The second example shows how computerized child health records have shown trends in measures of height and weight.[3] The Body Mass Index (weight in kilogrammes/height in metres^2) has increased over a

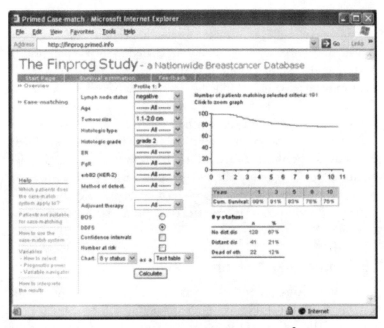

Fig. 7.1 Online estimation of prognosis with breast cancer[2].

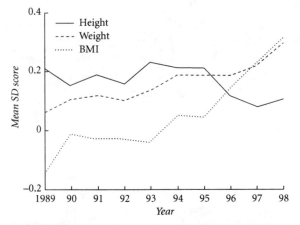

Fig. 7.2 Measures of height and weight in children[3]. Mean SD scores for weight, height and BMI plotted against year of measurement for children aged 2.9 to 4 years. Increasing trend in scores significant for weight and BMI but not for height.[3]

Note: Figures on this page reproduced with permission from the BMJ Publishing Group.

decade in children, partly due to an increase in weight and partly due to a reduction in height. If this reduction in height is real, and not a measurement artefact or a function of changing social composition of the population, this would be the first demonstration of a halt in the steady increase in childhood height which has been a feature of the second half of the twentieth century in Western countries. The authors make the point that 'routinely collected data are valuable in identifying anthropometric trends in populations'. Had we timely methods for monitoring such health trends in place, we might have identified the developing obesity epidemic earlier than we did and put preventive strategies in place—such strategies might have been easier to introduce, or more effective, at an earlier stage of the epidemic.

Electronic health records

The tremendous potential to answer public health questions, as clinical data are made available through the Electronic Health Record (EHR), is one of the major drivers of the move towards the EHR. This will not only enable large bodies of data to be captured and examined, but will enable this to be done quickly. If surveillance is to be useful, it has to report rapidly enough to allow reaction and intervention. If information is to be used for policy, it has to be timely to avoid making policy for tomorrow on the basis of information from yesterday (or yester year)—one of the criticisms of many disease registers!

Use of public health data

Public health exposures and outcomes are more complex than those acting at the individual level, as public health contextual influences on health have to be explored in addition to those acting at the level of the individual. For example, public health outcomes may be influenced by neighbourhood effects (see Chapter 2): public health and other intervention programmes, organizational issues of health services such as public/private financing of health and preventive services, contractual arrangements with practitioners and social and administrative service provision may all impact on health and need to be measured. These datasets are likely to be 'noisy' and unclean as they are usually collected for different purposes. To capture and analyse the complexity of such data requires computational power that e-science will be able to provide. Just thinking that providing a system for electronic health records will give us all we need to know and that this defines the limits of health informatics is a gross simplification.

Routinely-collected data may be able to be used to answer important public health questions, where a trial is not available. In the UK at present, there is a move to attempt to improve the care of patients with a number of conditions through the publication of National Service Frameworks (NSFs). Here, the Department of Health makes a number of demands of those who provide or organize patient care. The Coronary Heart Disease NSF, for example, requires each general practice to keep a register of all patients who have had a heart attack to monitor the use of secondary prevention agents. The opportunity to identify trends in treatment patterns, to link to outcome data and to examine how the two might be related is one that e-science could grasp. At the time of writing, however, there is no system for collecting and comparing relevant data. E-science should be able to offer help in answering the important public health questions for which the collection and analysis of timely and complex datasets are required.

One such example is in relation to the introduction of a new contract for general practitioners in the UK. Payment will be linked to the achievement of targets for treatment and preventive services. In the choice of targets, the evidence base was examined for evidence of effectiveness, but this was at the clinical effectiveness level. The opportunity to examine population effectiveness, across practices and wider administrative and geographic areas, can be gained by collecting and collating the data which will have to be processed to arrange for payments under the contract. An examination of the potential impact of the new contract on cardiovascular disease outcomes in a general practice population of 10,000 people,[4] is shown in Table 7.1. Future iterations of the contract might take the population perspective into account, and reward interventions more likely to have population than individual effectiveness and impact.

Table 7.1 Number of cardiovascular events prevented by the increased use of effective interventions (as proposed in a GP contract in the UK[4])

Intervention	Disease	Target proposed in GP contract	No of CVD events prevented over 5 year period
Cholesterol-lowering treatment	CHD*	60% ≤5.0	15.5
	Stroke	60% ≤5.0	7.2
	Diabetes	60% ≤5.0	6.5
Blood pressure lowering treatment	CHD	70% ≤150/90	3.6
	Stroke	70% ≤150/90	2.9
	Diabetes	55% ≤145/85	2.9
	Hypertension	70% ≤150/90	15.5
Aspirin	CHD*	90%	1.1
	Stroke	90%	0.4
ACE inhibitors/A2 antagonists	CHD and HF**	70%	1.2

*   CHD Coronary heart disease.
** HF Heart failure.

Use of administrative databases

It is possible to use data collected for administrative purposes to answer questions as suggested in relation to the GP contract above, and electronic administrative databases may be of use for public health decision-making.[5] Attention to the quality of the data is important: for example, co-morbidities appear to be widely underreported in Australian administrative databases.[6]

The importance of timeliness

None of the examples above have really utilized the major advantage of the new information technology, that of timeliness. Instant analysis is possible if data can be entered, checked and validated as soon as they are collected, offering the opportunity for speedy review and update of information. The CDC communicable disease surveillance system has recognized the value of this, but we have not yet fully realized the potential for other, less acute, public health problems. However, there is

> ## Box 7.1 Some tasks suited to Public Health informatics
>
> - Integration of complex datasets—exposures and outcomes—at the individual, population and organisational levels
> - Surveillance of trends in disease risk and outcomes including epidemics and bioterrorism
> - Timely production of health outcome data to allow integration of results into policy
> - Decision support systems to allow local data to be obtained and incorporated into policy.

no reason why the obesity epidemic could not have been spotted sooner and public health interventions put in place (and evaluated) to prevent this alarming trend.

Key summary points

- *The Student.* Public health informatics is: 'Knowledge, skills and tools for systematically creating information and managing knowledge to understand, protect and improve health in society.'
- *The Practitioner.* There are many opportunities to collect health service data and process them quickly so that lessons can be learned. The complexity of collecting and analysing public health exposures and outcomes in a timely fashion to feed into policy will only be realized by the use of electronic information-processing systems.
- *The Policy-maker.* Had routinely collected data on childhood height and weight been collected electronically and examined in a timely fashion, the obesity epidemic that is threatening large parts of the world could have been identified earlier and preventive policies put in place and evaluated.

References

1 Black N. and Payne M. Improving the use of clinical databases. *BMJ* 2002; **324**: 1194.

2   Lundin J., Lundin M., Isola J., Joensuu H. A web-based system for
    individualised survival estimation in breast cancer. *BMJ* 2003; **326**: 29.

3   Bundred P., Kitchiner D., Buchan I. Prevalence of overweight and obese
    children between 1989 and 1998: population-based series of cross-sectional
    studies. *BMJ* 2001; **322**: 326–8.

4   McElduff P., Lyratzopoulos G., Edwards R., Heller R. F., Shekelle P., Roland M.
    Will changes in primary care improve health outcomes? Modelling the
    impact of financial incentives introduced to improve quality of care in
    the UK. *Qual. Saf Health Care* 2004; **13**: 191–7.

5   Virnig B. A. and McBean M. Administrative data for public health
    surveillance and planning. *Annu. Rev. Public Health* 2001; **22**: 213–30.

6   Powell H., Lim L. L., Heller R. F. Accuracy of administrative data to assess
    comorbidity in patients with heart disease. an Australian perspective.
    J. Clin. Epidemiol. 2001; **54**: 687–93.

Part III

Understand and *use* the evidence

How can professionals and the public understand and use evidence to improve population health?

In Part II of this book, we saw how data can be collected. The next part of the evidence cycle asks us to understand and use that evidence: evidence into action. This involves risk perception, managing knowledge, and how to implement evidence in policy-making and prioritization. The section ends with tools for use in public health practice to support decision-making—Population impact assessment and Population health decision support.

Chapter 8

Perceptions of risk among policy-makers and the public

This chapter discusses how risk may be understood by, and communicated to, individuals, the 'public' and policy-makers.

Risk communication and public health

Most published work on risk perception and communication relates to the individual rather than to the central theme of this book, the population. Even where risks to public health are of concern, the approach has often centred on the individual. For example, there is a literature on how explaining risk to individuals will increase their uptake of a public health intervention such as screening or immunization. Let's start with immunization, where immunization may protect both the individual as well as the population—as a critical proportion of the population are required to be immunized to produce 'herd immunity'.

The publication of an hypothesis in 1998 in the *Lancet*, raised the spectre of a link between vaccination against measles, mumps and rubella (the MMR vaccine) and autism in children.[1] Despite the subsequent publication of numerous large studies which showed no such link, MMR vaccination rates started to fall—see Table 8.1—which contrasts with whooping cough vaccination with no fall. The reasons for this large dose of public misconception are not clear. Vaccination rates continued to fall in the face of reassurance from a number of professional bodies and the Department of Health. This was happening at a time of increasing scepticism and failure of public trust in the government in the UK.[2] Members of the medical profession were also

Table 8.1 Completed primary courses: percentage of children immunized by their second birthday, 1991–92 to 2001–02

	MMR	Whooping cough
1991–92	90	88
1992–93	92	91
1993–94	91	93
1994–95	91	93
1995–96	92	94
1996–97	92	94
1997–98	91	94
1998–99	88	94
1999–2000	88	94
2000–2001	87	94
2001–2002	84	93

NHS Immunisation Statistics, England: 2001–02
http://www.publications.doh.gov.uk/public/sb0218.xls

sceptical, and were sensitive to parental fears for their children.[3] It was suggested that given the setting in which most centrally decided health policy showed little regard for the collection or application of an evidence base, it was unrealistic for the Department of Health to expect health professionals to selectively respond to their interpretation of evidence in the MMR debate.[2]

Yet the failure of parents to vaccinate their children will produce a public health threat, as falling vaccination rates will be followed by outbreaks of the conditions they are designed to prevent. One of the most disappointing parts of this story is that those who are particularly concerned about the risks of MMR to their own children appear unlikely to respond to the knowledge that failure to vaccinate their children will lead to harm to others as herd immunity is reduced.[4] This illustrates the difficulties of extending from the individual to the population, and underlies the importance of developing methodologies that will allow an understanding of risks and benefits at the population level.

There is a literature on the methods of individualizing risk to increase another public health intervention, that of screening. A systematic review has found that individualized risk communication (using specific risk estimates for individuals) leads to increased participation in screening programmes.[5] While this is a strategy that might be beneficial for public health, this result is not due to an appropriate understanding of a public health benefit. How we communicate benefits to the community rather than to individuals appears to be a major difficulty.

While Calman, who was England's Chief Medical Officer in the 1990s, has differentiated between individual and public risk communication, his demonstrations of simple ways of presenting risk are targeted at individuals rather than the population risks and benefits.[6] There have been a number of studies on ways of communicating risk in pictorial or other mechanisms to individuals.[7] There has also been a suggestion that patient choice modules could be presented that would help patients to make evidence-based choices.[8] A UK Department of Health report identified two main perspectives:[9] one reflects empirical research on reactions to risk, while the second considers risk communication as a decision process. The aim of the report was to provide 'pointers to good practice' based on well-established research that can be adapted to individual circumstances.

The framing and presentation of risk

There are large amounts of data which suggest that the way measures of risk are framed or communicated has an influence on the actions taken. This has mainly been studied in terms of doctors giving advice to patients. Some studies have looked at the actions policy-makers would take based on the presentation of risk estimates. The general finding is that people find relative risk to be more appealing than absolute risk.[10] Drug companies have been capitalizing on this for a long time and tend to use relative risk in their advertising.[10] Despite the frequent demonstration of the preference among those surveyed for relative over absolute presentations of risk, a systematic review concluded that a number of factors reduced the impact of framing—such as the risk of causing harm, the presence of pre-existing prejudices about treatments, the type of decision, the therapeutic yield, clinical experience and costs.[11] The authors further made the point that none of the studies had investigated the effect of framing on actual clinical practice.

Note on the difference between relative and absolute risk

The importance of the use of absolute measures of risk and benefit has been a recurring theme of this book and underlies much of the derivation of population impact measures for interventions in Chapter 4. Let's imagine a treatment that cuts risk of death from 10 in every 100 patients to 5 in every 100. We could say that, relative to the rate before treatment, the death rate is halved. This is what we mean by relative risk. In absolute terms, five people in every 100 still die, even with treatment, so we refer to this risk as the absolute risk. It, too, in this example is five in 100, the same as the relative risk.

However, this is not invariable! Let's suppose the treatment cuts deaths by one half, but the condition only leads to 10 deaths in 10,000 patients. The relative risk—relating the risk with treatment to that without treatment—remains the same as in the first example: it is 50%. In absolute terms, however, the risk goes down from 10 in 10,000 to 5 in 10,000.

Put the two examples together. In the first, the absolute risk was originally one in 10. With treatment it was halved and the relative risk—with to without treatment—was 50%. In the second example, the same relative risk applied but an absolute risk that was small anyway—one in 1,000—simply became slightly lower; one in 5,000.

When you ponder the two ways of presenting risk, especially changes in risk that may follow from treatment, you can see just how different perceptions will be if you say 'reduced relative risk by half' or 'reduced absolute risk by half'! This is a very simplistic expression of the relative versus absolute risk debate, which has been more extensively discussed in Chapter 4. The implications of the different expressions of risk and benefit are quite different. Angell and Kassirer express this well in relation to a large trial of two drugs to reduce deaths after heart attacks:[12]

> For example, the results of the GUSTO trial could be framed in three ways:
> t-PA was 14 percent more effective than streptokinase; t-PA lowered the

mortality from 7.3 percent to 6.3 percent; or t-PA increased the survival rate from 92.7 percent to 93.7 percent. All three ways are accurate, but they produce very different impressions on readers.

Communicating risk to health policy-makers

Evidence-based health policy making depends on the appropriate understanding of risks and benefits of different policy options. Health policy is made by physicians (usually at the micro level) and by those in positions to allocate resources (often working in health departments at local or government levels). Both would be expected to have a good understanding of risk and benefit when making their decisions. There have been few examinations of the impact of framing on health policy decision-making, although one landmark paper by Fahey and colleagues showed that policy-makers would be more likely to fund programmes (mammography and cardiac rehabilitation) on the basis of benefit presented as relative risk than absolute risk reductions.[13] As in the conclusion of the systematic review above, this was a theoretical exercise, and the results may well not be reflected in real life. The drivers of health policy decision-making may well be much more extensive than just an appreciation of risk and benefit among the decision-makers—this is discussed more fully in Chapter 10.

Theory of risk communication

Risk may be defined as the probability of the occurrence of an undesirable outcome. There have been a number of theories of risk: Ulrich Beck, in his book *Risk Society* suggests that risks are produced by socially and industrially determined factors:[14] Mary Douglas, in her 'cultural theory of risk' suggests that risk perception is influenced by cultural values and beliefs, which influence risk-taking and risk avoidance.[15] A number of medical commentators have tried to develop a pragmatic approach to risk, in order to help us communicate risk appropriately.

Bennett's document on communicating risks identifies a number of theoretical aspects of risk appreciation in relation to public health, and is well worth reading.[9] Amongst other issues, he has identified a number of features of risk that invoke public concern. He says that risk is more worrying if it:

- is involuntary rather than voluntary
- threatens a form of death, illness or injury which arouses particular dread
- damages identifiable victims
- is poorly understood by science
- is subject to contradictory statements from responsible sources or from the same source
- is inequitably distributed
- is inescapable
- arises from an unfamiliar or novel source
- results from man-made rather than natural sources
- causes hidden and irreversible damage
- poses particular danger to small children, pregnant women or future generations.

The role of the media

The media has a role to play in the way the public is presented with information on risk.

An excellent study has examined the coverage by the news media of the benefits and risks of medications and found a number of inadequacies in reporting, including excessive focus on relative risk reductions.[16] Among the 60 per cent of stories that quantified the benefits at all, the vast majority used relative rather than absolute benefits.

There is little research on the understanding of risk by the public. Media reports are important ways for the public to appreciate the risks of public health interventions. It is likely that reporters are poorly informed about the different ways and implications of expressing risk. However, in the UK, the Guild of Health Writers has taken an initiative to improve the knowledge of health reporters, and the Royal Media Society has produced a report for both scientists and the media about best practice in communicating risk[17] (http://www.royalsoc.ac.uk/files/statfiles/document-161.pdf).

An extensive Kings Fund Report[18] has documented a number of health scares raised by the media. It found that a number of health policy-makers who were interviewed for the report were concerned about the discrepancy between the importance of the public health risks and the news coverage given. The role of the media is not necessarily to improve public health—it is to interest individuals enough for them to access the media product. We certainly need to find ways of helping the media to report health risks and benefits in ways that will help, not hinder, an improvement in public health.

Population health decision support

Whether for the media, for individuals, or for policy-makers at the clinical or population level, help is needed. The final chapter in this book offers the concept of 'Population health decision support'—a method of helping policy-makers appreciate population level risks and benefits to help with prioritizing health interventions.

Key summary points

◆ *The Student.* Although there has been much written about the perception and communication of risk, this has mainly related to individuals. The communication of risk about populations has special problems and issues.

◆ *The Practitioner.* There are various theories of risk communication, some of which may be of use in communicating population risk to improve the health of the population. The media has a special responsibility for communicating risk relating to public health issues, but finds individual risk more appealing to its customers.

◆ *The Policy-maker.* Using individual risk communication methods to improve population health is often inappropriate. The incorporation of population health outcomes and values should not be ignored when risk communication is considered.

References

1   Horton R. The lessons of MMR. *Lancet* 2004; **363**: 747–9.
2   Heller R. F. and Heller T. A failure of public trust. *Practitioner* 2002; **246**: 511.
3   Heller T. Ethical debate: Vaccination against mumps, measles, and rubella: is there a case for deepening the debate? How safe is MMR vaccine? *BMJ* 2001; **323**: 838–9.

4 Heller D., Heller T., Patison S. MMR vaccine debate: authors' summary of responses. *BMJ* 2002; **324**: 733.

5 Edwards A., Unigwe S., Elwyn G., Hood K. Effects of communicating individual risks in screening programmes: Cochrane systematic review. *BMJ* 2003; **327**: 703–9.

6 Calman K. C. Communication of risk: choice, consent, and trust. *Lancet* 2002; **360**: 166–8.

7 Edwards A., Elwyn G., Mulley A. Explaining risks: turning numerical data into meaningful pictures. *BMJ* 2002; **324**: 827–30.

8 Holmes-Rovner M., Llewellyn-Thomas H., Entwistle V., Coulter A., O'Connor A., Rovner D. R. Patient choice modules for summaries of clinical effectiveness: a proposal. *BMJ* 2001; **322**: 664–7.

9 Department of Health. *Communicating about risks to Public Health: Pointers to Good Practice.* London: UK Department of Health, 1998.

10 Skolbekken J. A. Communicating the risk reduction achieved by cholesterol reducing drugs. *BMJ* 1998; **316**: 1956–8.

11 McGettigan P., Sly K., O'Connell D., Hill S., Henry D. The effects of information framing on the practices of physicians. *Journal of General Internal Medicine* 1999; **14**: 633–42.

12 Angell M. and Kassirer J. P. Clinical research—what should the public believe? *N. Engl. J. Med.* 1994; **331**: 189–90.

13 Fahey T., Griffiths S., Peters T. J. Evidence-based purchasing: understanding results of clinical trials and systematic reviews. *BMJ* 1995; **311**: 1056–9.

14 Beck U. *Risk Society:towards a new modernity.* Translated by Mark Ritter. London: Sage, 1992.

15 Douglas M. *Risk and Blame: essays in cultural theory.* London: Routledge, 1992.

16 Moynihan R., Bero L., Ross-Degnan D., Henry D., Lee K., Watkins J., *et al.* Coverage by the news media of the benefits and risks of medications. *N. Engl. J. Med.* 2000; **342**: 1645–50.

17 Social Issues Research Centre. *Guidelines on Science and Health Communication.* Oxford: Social Issues Research Centre, 2001.

18 Harrabin R., Coote A., Allen J. *Health in the News: Risk, reporting and media influence.* London: Kings Fund Publications, 2003.

Chapter 9

Managing knowledge for population health

This chapter looks at how we can turn data into knowledge that can be used to implement the collected evidence—evidence into action.

Evidence-based medicine (EBM) has taught us that we need to think of how to access, appraise and apply health evidence. One of the most impressive cornerstones of EBM has been the work on providing access to the research literature. The revolution in library searching techniques and computerized access has been fundamental. Critical appraisal has been a fundamental skill taught to clinicians in many settings and the method of synthesizing evidence embodied by the Cochrane Collaboration and others has made a major contribution. Most of this relates to published research literature, and before we can apply this to public health practice, we need to think of what other sources of evidence might be available. We are likely going to have to broaden our activities in the areas of access and appraisal before we can apply evidence in the public health field. We have already discussed that the usual research hierarchy and reliance on the randomized controlled trial, as being mainstays of EBM, may not be sufficient for evidence for population health.

We can think about a taxonomy that might help. Data, which may comprise numbers of pieces of observation, can become information if it is accessed and assembled properly. When this information is going to be used for something, it becomes knowledge, but it has to be appraised first.

Data might be observations that are collected as part of routine processes of care or management, or they might be collected as part of a research exercise, or they might come from experience. You will

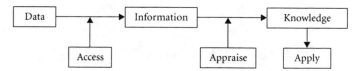

Fig. 9.1 The process of turning data into knowledge which can be applied.

remember that our definition of Pubic Health pays due recognition to experience as an important part of the evidence base. Muir Gray, one of the earliest advocates for an evidence base in public health, defines *research, data* and *experience* as the three levels of knowledge required to build an evidence base for use in public health (Faculty of Public Health Annual Conference, 2002).

There is another strand of definitions of knowledge to fit into this schema. We have been talking so far about explicit knowledge, that is, knowledge derived from external sources. But there is also tacit knowledge, which is mainly experience-based. The importance of acknowledging this is that tacit knowledge needs to be incorporated into the evidence base appropriately and turned into explicit knowledge that the individual or organization can use.[1]

Levels of knowledge

Research

The incorporation of knowledge derived from research into policy is discussed in Chapter 10, and is central to our theme of evidence for population health. An interesting paper published in 2001 is one of a number of attempts to explore the potential of research to impact on the provision of health services.[2] Public health practitioners in Norway had a positive attitude towards research-based information, but did not think that such information would really help them solve problems. They conclude: 'There is an unrealised potential in public health practice for more frequent and extensive use of research-based information.'

Data

In Chapter 7 we discussed how there are many unused pieces of data which exist in the health arena and how e-science might come to our rescue in both collecting and interpreting them. There are, however, a number of routinely collected sources of health data which are available for scrutiny by health professionals or the public. These have been discussed previously in terms of health outcome measures, and we do not need to repeat them here.

We should also consider how data can help the assessment of the broader determinants of health. Saunders *et al.* have listed a number of types of data which are relevant in the UK.[3] These are physical environment; crime; housing and homelessness; social services; socio-economic environment including employment; lifestyle; education; leisure and culture; transport; accidents. A number of non-medical data sets are available to examine these areas, and these are nicely documented in the paper quoted above.

Each country will have their own sets of these data, and there are also international collections, such as from the World Health Organization through routine statistical collections or the World Health Report, which identifies particular issues. We have touched on a number of these in previous chapters. In the UK, and in parts of Europe, the Public Health Observatories play an important role in making data available online. They have been criticized for focusing on the data aspects and not developing a knowledge (intelligence) function, to help the data be used. Having read this chapter, it is clear that we need to do more than collect data. We need the next steps to ensure that they are used. A number of electronic sources of data are available, and for the UK, the National Electronic Library of Health (http://www.nelh.nhs.uk/) is an excellent resource—with links to a number of sites including the Office for National Statistics.

The use of data bases that are collected for routine care have been identified as potentially valuable sources of data to examine health outcomes. High quality clinical databases can be found on an extensive and helpful web site.[4]

As we have discussed in our paper, 'A population focus to evidence-based medicine: evidence for population health', data at both the individual and population levels are important in building the evidence base for public health.[5]

Tacit knowledge also offers data—such data are usually inside the heads of those who have had the experience to provide the knowledge, and not available unless through the medium of discussions and presentations.

Experience

Muir Gray, again, has described how knowledge can be mobilized from experience. Tacit knowledge can be enhanced to become explicit knowledge by the use of published information. Explicit knowledge can be enriched by reuse. We should not forget the importance of experience, but should remember that it can be assisted and enhanced. This tacit knowledge can be at both the individual and the collective (or population) levels. Ethnographers have many examples of cultural knowledge which may never be written, but which shapes the health behaviour of populations. In the context of a health impact assessment of a proposed diamond mining project in northern Canada, 'traditional knowledge' was assessed, which they defined as 'the knowledge, innovations and practices of indigenous and/or local communities developed from experience gained over the centuries and adapted to local culture and environment'.[6] Acceptance of immunization against measles is another example of the importance of understanding public perceptions and cultural beliefs.[7] If we are going to help populations to improve their health, we are going to have to incorporate tacit knowledge such as these examples, and not rely totally on evidence from randomized controlled trials!

Managing the knowledge

Knowledge management has recently become a recognizable term. It has been defined as a structured process that enables knowledge to be *created, stored, distributed* and *applied* to decision-making.[1] We have discussed the creation of different types of knowledge above. How this knowledge may be stored is also touched on in the e-science chapter, and the revolution in information and communication technology will allow many advances in future years. Libraries have been the traditional methods of storing knowledge, and tacit knowledge is stored in peoples' brains. The distribution of knowledge is also helped by the revolution in information and communication technology, as evidenced by the use of the Internet. How to distribute tacit knowledge from peoples' brains is potentially more difficult for an organization that wishes to benefit from such knowledge. The application of knowledge so that it can be used for problem solving and decision-making is central to the implementation of evidence into practice.

Table 9.1 shows how using the principles of knowledge management could be of value.

This brings us into a large territory of behaviour change, and in terms of application of knowledge in a health setting, we do need to consider if both tacit and explicit knowledge are appropriately integrated and made available to those who are expected to implement

Table 9.1 How the principles of knowledge management can be applied Example: general practitioners are not familiar with data on the baseline risk of health outcomes, nor of current practice levels: interpreting the impact of a proposed intervention on their practice population depends on this knowledge

Principles of knowledge management	The problem	Possible solutions
Generation	Explicit, local data are not generated on current practice levels, or on health outcomes for patient groups of different ages. Tacit knowledge currently used	Data on patient groups entered onto disease registers and linked to health outcomes through hospital and mortality data—electronic health records would assist
Storage	No way of storing data on current practice and health outcomes. Tacit knowledge, stored in minds and practice 'ethos' currently used, but not able to be shared	Registers will allow a way of storing and releasing data, allowing for confidentiality
Distribution	No way of distributing such knowledge to GPs, other than guidelines which do not have local context and which usually do not have a population focus	Web-based systems could be used as a repository for the register data above, and made available— in anonymized form to protect confidentiality
Application	No current way of helping GPs to prioritize between alternative interventions on the basis of population impact at point of decision-making	Decision support systems, again web-based, would allow local context to be applied

evidence. The failure of many practice guidelines to be implemented effectively[8] is a testament to this difficulty. Chapter 12 is an attempt to offer support for the implementation of population health decision-making, and does attempt to integrate explicit and tacit knowledge (although on reflection, we have certainly focused heavily on explicit knowledge!).

Within an organization, the critical factors for ensuring adequate knowledge management have been said to be leadership, use of information and communication technology, the organizational culture and the development of skills capacity for the workforce.[1] These factors will apply generally, and are not specific to organizations that work in public health.

Key summary points

♦ *The Student.* Data need to be accessed appropriately so that they can become information, which needs to be critically appraised before it becomes knowledge. Knowledge may be explicit (based on external sources) or tacit (based on experience).

♦ *The Practitioner.* Knowledge may come from data sources (of which a number are available and a number exist but are difficult to access), research or experience.

♦ *The Policy-maker.* Organizational issues that allow knowledge to be managed (and turned into practice) include leadership, use of information and communication technology, the organizational culture and the development of skills capacity for the workforce.

References

1 Sandars J. Knowledge management: something old, something new! *Work Based Learning in Primary Care* 2004; **2**: 9–17.

2 Forsetlund L. and Bjorndal A. The potential for research-based information in public health: identifying unrecognised information needs. *BMC. Public Health* 2001; **1**: 1.

3 Saunders P., Mathers J., Parry J., Stevens A. Identifying 'non-medical' datasets to monitor community health and well-being. *J. Public Health Med.* 2001; **23**: 103–8.

4 Black N. and Payne M. Improving the use of clinical databases. *BMJ* 2002; **324**: 1194.

5   Heller R. F. and Page J. H. A population perspective to evidence-based medicine: 'evidence for population health'. *Journal of Epidemiology and Community Health* 2002; **56**: 45–7.

6   Kwiatkowski R. E. and Ooi M. Integrated environmental impact assessment: a Canadian example. *Bull. World Health Organ* 2003; **81**: 434–8.

7   Serquina-Ramiro L., Kasniyah N., Inthusoma T., Higginbotham N., Streiner D., Nichter M., *et al.* Measles immunization acceptance in Southeast Asia: past patterns and future challenges. *Southeast Asian J. Trop. Med. Public Health* 2001; **32**: 791–804.

8   Grimshaw J. M., Shirran L., Thomas R., Mowatt G., Fraser C., Bero L., *et al.* Changing provider behavior: an overview of systematic reviews of interventions. *Med. Care* 2001; **39**: 112–45.

Chapter 10

Applying evidence to inform public health practice and health policy decision-making

This chapter discusses the tensions between the health evidence base and other factors in making prioritization decisions that will influence public health and its practice.

General issues in setting priorities for population health

The need for priority setting in the field of health care comes from the reality that the demand for health care exceeds the availability of resources. This excess is clearly different in different settings, but the problem is getting worse everywhere, due partly to the ageing of the population and the increasing availability of new (and expensive) technologies, including medications. How the need for health care can be balanced with the need for improving the health of the community through means other than health care is a particular issue of interest to population health.

We have spent much of the book examining the evidence base for population health. However, the implementation of evidence into policy is in many ways more difficult than just collecting the evidence, and has not been tackled in as systematic a way. I have drawn on the work of a number of authors to develop this schema, resulting in Figure 10.1, which has the form of a balance between the two drivers of the policy-making process. Rychetnick and colleagues[1] have offered a useful classification, which I have used as a basis for describing the balance between rigorous appraisal of the evidence (as per our

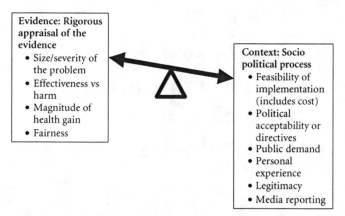

Fig. 10.1 The balance between evidence and context—rigorous appraisal of the evidence and the sociopolitical processes that go into policy decision-making for implementing an intervention.

discussion of levels of evidence in Chapter 5) and the sociopolitical process that are also crucial to implementation of policy. Bhopal, in his excellent book *Concepts of Epidemiology* identifies two major drivers to priority setting—scientific and social/political/economic.[2] The same distinction is nicely encapsulated by Dobrow and colleagues who identify 'evidence' and 'context' axes for decision-making.[3] They show how the evidence-based medicine movement rates highly on the 'evidence' scale, but low on the 'context' scale. Singer identifies fairness and legitimacy (who should have the authority to make decisions),[4] which also map onto the two drivers, which seem to revolve around the evidence and the context. I have added some points made by Elliott and Popay, who described some of the barriers to evidence-based decision-making,[5] in drawing the figure. You can see which way I have tilted the balance!

Rosenstock and Lee comment on ways of responding to the threats to obtaining evidence in a way that will lead to its incorporation into policy:[6]

> Maintaining the capacity for evidence-based policy requires differentiating between honest scientific challenge and evident vested interest and responding accordingly, building and diversifying partnerships, assuring the transparency of funding sources, agreeing on rules for publication, and distinguishing the point where science ends and policy begins.

As we develop evidence for population health, we must ensure that the context in which decisions are made is fully understood as crucial to the implementation of evidence into public health practice. The quantification of costs and health gain may play only a small part in the decision-making process. I think that this is partly due to the poor methods currently available for estimating and comparing health gains to the population. It is one of my missions to show how health gain can be assessed at the population level so that it plays a more important role in decision-making.

Collecting the evidence

Returning to the 'collect' part of the Population Health Evidence Cycle, there is now increasing recognition that the way the evidence is generated in the first place will have an impact on how it is utilized. Research priorities have to be set, and these should not only reflect the interest of the researcher, but the values of the users of the

Table 10.1 Combined approach matrix for priority setting

Five steps in priority setting	Actors/factors determining the health status of a population (intervention levels)				
	Global level	Individual, family and community level	Level of health ministry, health research institutions, health systems and services	Level of sectors other than health	Level of central government
1. Level of disease burden					
2. Determinants for persistence					
3. Present level of knowledge					
4. Cost-effectiveness of future interventions					
5. Resource flows					

From the Global Forum on Health Research (http://www.globalforumhealth.org).

research. Lomas and colleagues identify two main approaches to setting research priorities as 'technical' and 'interpretive': the latter can use their 'listening model' for involving stakeholders at various stages of the priority-setting process.[7]

Those of us who work in high income health economies have a great deal to learn from those in low to middle income economies in many ways, including how to set priorities. Where resources are limited, the imperative to spend the small amount available in the most effective way is greater than where we are playing at the margins of health gain. The Global Forum on Health Research is the latest in a distinguished line of initiatives to help low income economies to identify disease burden and health care and prevention priorities. This arises from the identification of the '10/90 gap'—only about 10 per cent of health research funds from public and private sources are devoted to 90 per cent of the world's health problems. The Global Forum has encouraged use of the 'combined approach matrix' which brings together in a systematic framework all current knowledge related to a particular disease or risk factor, and relates the 'five steps in priority setting' (an economic axis) to those who can make decisions on the health status of a population the 'actors and factors' (Table 10.1). This model can be used in a number of health settings.

The size of the problem

Part of the rigorous appraisal of the evidence involves making an assessment of the size of the problem and the potential benefits of the new policy. In Chapter 4, we spent some time discussing how we can measure the burden of disease and the population impact of interventions and disease causation. We will, in fact, come back to this in the final chapter with a toolkit for assessing the population impact. There have been many attempts to measure the burden of illness, but one is worth picking out here as it is designed to be directly relevant to policy making for preventive services. Coffield and colleagues designed a method to compare the value of clinical preventive services.[8] They ranked these services on the basis of the 'clinically preventable burden' and the cost-effectiveness, using the quality adjusted life year (QALY) as the main outcome measure. They calculated a score from 0 to 10 for each potential service, and found a number which scored highly, are delivered to 50 per cent or less of the target population, and are important missed opportunities for preventing disease and promoting health. We have previously discussed the different ways of assessing cost-effectiveness, and the limitations of the QALY as a measure of use to population health decision-making. Despite these limitations, this combination of the QALY and other ways of providing a ranking offers considerable potential for determining policy priorities.

A debate took place in the pages of the *BMJ* that nicely captured the issue of evidence and public policy. A group, which included the editors of the Lancet and BMJ, blamed a UK government inquiry into health inequalities of lacking an evidence base for its recommendations.[9] A commentary provided a counterpoint, that for a number of public health interventions (including many of those which might help to reduce health inequalities) the evidence base just was not available.[10]

Back to implementation

Whatever methods of measuring the burden of illness are chosen there is an issue of identifying need in terms that can be related to a defined population and in a way that can be fed into identifying priorities and then into decision-making. The pathway described below, where the measurement of the disease burden leads to some action such as commissioning of services, is the ideal.

The challenge is not only to make sure that the measurement of the disease burden is appropriate, but that systems are in place to follow the path to lead to action, and that effective interventions are available to be commissioned.

The debate continues

Some have argued that there are limits to the value of evidence in policy-making,[11] others respond that research is essential to

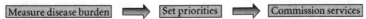

Fig. 10.2 From measurement to commissioning.

contribute to health policy-making[12] and that it is also possible to apply evidence to policy and management![13,14]

I can't claim to have the answer to all this, but this chapter should serve to indicate the debate and some of the parameters for thinking about this important issue. Singer has an excellent quote suggesting that more work is required:

> The pressing research challenge is to develop and evaluate an interdisciplinary methodology for resource allocation decision making that incorporates but goes beyond EBM (Evidence-Based Medicine) and CEA (Cost-Effectiveness Analysis); integrates the various theoretical approaches to resource allocation of philosophy, law, political science, economics, and clinical epidemiology; proves useful to resource allocation decision makers; and is perceived as fair by the communities whose resources are at stake.[15]

Key summary points

◆ *The Student.* The implementation of evidence into policy is driven by two balancing themes—the rigour of the evidence and the sociopolitical decision-making process.

◆ *The Practitioner.* The way in which stakeholders are listened to and involved in designing the research will be important in how the results are implemented.

◆ *The Policy-maker.* There is a challenge to develop better methods of incorporating evidence into health priority setting.

References

1 Rychetnik L., Frommer M., Hawe P., Shiell A. Criteria for evaluating evidence on public health interventions. *J. Epidemiol. Community Health* 2002; **56**: 119–27.

2 Bhopal R. *Concepts of Epidemiology: an integrated introduction to the ideas, theories, principles and methods of epidemiology.* Oxford: Oxford University Press, 2002.

3 Dobrow M. J., Goel V., Upshur R. E. Evidence-based health policy: context and utilisation. *Soc. Sci. Med.* 2004; **58**: 207–17.

4 Singer P. A., Martin D. K., Giacomini M., Purdy L. Priority setting for new technologies in medicine: qualitative case study. *BMJ* 2000; **321**: 1316–18.

5 Elliott H., Popay J. How are policy makers using evidence? Models of research utilisation and local NHS policy making. *J. Epidemiol. Community Health* 2000; **54**: 461–8.

6 Rosenstock L. and Lee L. J. Attacks on science: the risks to evidence-based policy. *Am. J. Public Health* 2002; **92**: 14–18.

7 Lomas J., Fulop N., Gagnon D., Allen P. On being a good listener: setting priorities for applied health services research. *Milbank Q.* 2003; **81**:.363–88.

8 Coffield A. B., Maciosek M. V., McGinnis J. M., Harris J. R., Caldwell M. B., Teutsch S. M. *et al*. Priorities among recommended clinical preventive services. *Am. J. Prev. Med.* 2001; **21**: 1–9.

9 Macintyre S., Chalmers I., Horton R., Smith R. Using evidence to inform health policy: case study. *BMJ* 2001; **322**: 222–5.

10 Davey S. G., Ebrahim S., Frankel S. How policy informs the evidence. *BMJ* 2001; **322**: 184–5.

11 Black N. Evidence-based policy: proceed with care. *BMJ* 2001; **323**: 275–9.

12 Donald A. Commentary: research must be taken seriously. *BMJ* 2001; **323**: 278–9.

13 Walshe K. Evidence-based policy: don't be timid. *BMJ* 2001; **323**: 1187.

14 Walshe K. and Rundall T. G. Evidence-based management: from theory to practice in health care. *Milbank Q.* 2001; **79**: 429–57.

15 Singer P. A. Resource allocation: beyond evidence-based medicine and cost-effectiveness analysis. *ACP J. Club.* 1997; **127**: A16–18.

Chapter 11

Individual or population priorities for population health: involving the public

This chapter discusses how there are differences between individual and population health priorities, how the Population Evidence Cycle may offer an organizing structure for how to involve the public in priority setting, and provides a new definition of public health which acknowledges the importance of the public.

The individual or the population?

Margaret Thatcher is supposed to have said that there is no such thing as a population, it is just a collection of individuals and families. In setting health priorities, what benefits an individual or a family may create tensions at the population level. The example of people not allowing their children to be vaccinated against a communicable disease is an extreme illustration of this, as it may put others in the population at risk. The funding of an expensive facility which benefits a small number of individuals, may adversely affect the funding of something that would benefit more people in the community. We can classify the questions that this raises as follows:[1,2]

Questions that arise in judging benefits to the individual and the community

Judging the benefit to the individual

- ◆ How large is the possible benefit to the individual?
- ◆ What is the cost, and on whom does it fall?
- ◆ Does the benefit outweigh the cost for the individual?

Judging the benefit to the community

+ How large is the possible benefit to the population?

+ What are alternative uses of resources for a similar or greater benefit?

+ How does one make the choice?

Chapter 4 shows how we can go from measures of benefit that apply at the individual level to those that apply at the population level.

I have bemoaned the fact, in Chapter 5, that while we have good evidence for the benefits of pharmaceutical agents, we have less good evidence for population-based interventions, largely due to the financial stimulus of the pharmaceutical industry to support trials of their products. We don't have similar trials of community-based interventions. We don't know either if pharmaceutical or other interventions would be more effective at reducing the social gradient for diseases such as heart disease.

> The tendency for those who need preventive care the least to seek it the most is one of the weaknesses of taking a one-at-a-time approach to patient care. There are 3 levels of thinking and action: treating individuals purely as individuals, treating them as members of a group, and treating communities without specific attention to the individuals within them. For physicians, the distinction is between acting in the public interest on a succession of persons versus intervening on communities—as with radio and television advertisements and community campaigns. . . . Certainly the large amount of money spent on medication . . . is not matched by spending on community-based or public health initiatives that may well have a similar or greater effect.[2]

The fundamental thesis of this book is that we need methods to develop and implement an evidence base for population health decisions. The emphasis on individual-level drivers of decision-making is even accentuated by the difficulties in involving the public in decision-making. I'd now like to discuss how we can bring the public back into public health.

Putting the public back into public health

Although the public, or the population, are ostensibly the target group of public health activity, they are in general not consulted or involved in decision-making about the health of the public. The public do not seek care or prevention in the way that sick individuals do. Those responsible for the health of the public do not even include the public in their definition of public health. The UK Faculty of Public Health uses a definition coined by the Acheson Committee on Public Health as: 'The science and art of preventing disease, prolonging life and promoting health through organised efforts of society.'

In the UK, the Commission for Patient and Public Involvement in Health was set up in January 2003. It is an independent, non-departmental public body, sponsored by the Department of Health. Its remit is to ensure that the public is involved in decision-making about health and health services. The UK Department of Health has established legislation (in 2003) for patients' forums (to be known as Patient and Public Involvement (PPI) Forums) for each hospital trust and Primary Care Trust across England. Individuals nominate themselves, will include patients or patient support group members. The Department of Health website, http://www.cppih.org/ says nothing about public health in any of the discussions about public involvement: it is all to do with patients.

The most famous attempt to involve the public in decisions about public health priority setting was the Oregon Health Plan. Initially developed in 1987 and passed by the Oregon legislature in 1989, planners prioritized those services for which the state would pay under Oregon's Medicaid programme. A prioritized list of health services that would be covered under the plan was developed through a communal process of public hearings, community meetings, and telephone surveys. The Health Services Commission, following many hours of public hearings around the state, established a prioritized list of more than 700 physical health, dental, chemical dependency and mental health services. The legislature sets the funding level to cover a certain number of services on the list, but cannot rearrange the list (see http://www.dhs.state.or.us/healthplan/priorlist/history.html).

The Plan was criticized as not having obtained appropriate and fully informed preferences from the population. We have seen as a common theme in this book how difficult it is to establish the true health gain for a population—Chapter 12 will provide a decision-support system to help planners, but the methods are still under development. It is even more complicated when trying to ensure that public perceptions of health gain are accurate. There are a number of methodological considerations about how the public's views on priority setting can be obtained, for example Dolan and colleagues have shown that priorities assigned by members of the public changed after they had the chance to discuss them.[3]

Getting the definition right

With all the difficulties discussed above, at least if we get the definition of public health to include reference to the public it would be a start. An alternative definition of public health[4] meets the objective of including the public:

> Use of theory, experience and evidence derived through the population sciences to improve the health of the population in a way that best meets the implicit and explicit needs of the community (the public).

Making public health accountable to the public

As we have seen above, there are some attempts to involve the public, although these are mostly for individual patient decision-making. It might be useful to consider this through the Population Health Evidence Cycle,[5] where we can see at which points of the cycle the public can be involved.

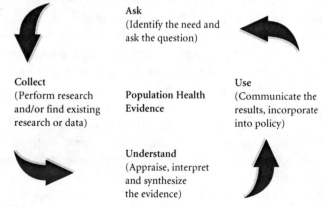

Ask
(Identify the need and ask the question)

Collect
(Perform research and/or find existing research or data)

Population Health Evidence

Use
(Communicate the results, incorporate into policy)

Understand
(Appraise, interpret and synthesize the evidence)

Fig. 11.1 The Population Health Evidence cycle[5].

Ask for the evidence

I am not sure who can be the 'conscience' of the public in terms of demanding appropriate levels of public health. Governments are elected on the basis that they promise what they think the public wants, but their interpretation of public wishes is not particularly sophisticated! Much health policy seems to regard short waiting times for medical attention and hospital admission as the most important way of meeting public demand for health care. Most public representation on one of the world's most advanced systems for 'consumer' involvement is the Consumers' Health Forum of Australia— http://www.chf.org.au/index.asp. Although an increasing number of Australian government committees now include a consumer representative, they are often a lone voice with limited expert knowledge and require resources and support to ensure that they ask the right questions and provide a true 'public' input. This is a common issue in whatever country consumer input is accepted. There does not seem to be an easy method for the public to ask the question of whether true population priorities are being met by the health service. When we go beyond health services to issues such as adequate attention to environmental or societal factors that influence public health, there is no clear forum, let alone public voice. Who is taking the public's public health needs into account, to avoid the development of childhood obesity? Does 'the public' have a view on this? If so, what is it? Maybe the readers of this book can answer some of the questions.

Collect the evidence

Rapid appraisal is an excellent example of how the needs and views of the public can be used for health planning, and Murray offers a number of interesting examples of how this technique can be used.[6] It is of relevance in a number of international settings. These and other more formal methods are available for assessing community views. Again, the initiative appears to come mainly from the health professionals rather than from the public themselves, and are usually task-specific (although one of the examples given by Murray did lead to the establishment of an ongoing health forum).

Understand the evidence

There are a number of examples of educational exercises for the public to help them understand and critically appraise evidence. Many of these examples are related to specific diseases: one notable example is Kay Dickerson's short course in critical appraisal for breast cancer patients to help them understand their illness. Patient choice modules for summaries of clinical effectiveness have been proposed. We have discussed risk communication above (Chapter 8). The understanding of population risk and the appreciation of risks to the community of individual action (such as choice not to have children immunized) require sophisticated knowledge.

Use the evidence

We are back to public involvement in the decision-making process itself at this point in the Population Health Evidence Cycle. The public may feel remote from effective entry into the decision-making process,[5] and as suggested above, may be ineffectual even if offered token involvement in such decision-making. If evidence is not used in health policy-making, the views of the public are not likely to be used either.

Conclusion

The proposed definition of public health and the framework afforded by the Population Health Evidence Cycle might help focus attention on the need for, and methods by which, the public can engage with public health. Putting the public back into public health is not going to be easy, but should be attempted. If we are to attempt to make health policy decisions that favour population level health impacts, such a goal is essential.

Key summary points

+ *The Student.* Use of the evidence cycle can help identify how population health policy decision-making can be accountable to the public.

- *The Practitioner.* A new definition of public health is advocated:
  Use of theory, experience and evidence derived through the population sciences to improve the health of the population in a way that best meets the implicit and explicit needs of the community (the public).

- *The Policy-maker.* Different levels of decision-making are required to impact on the individual and the population. We need to find better ways of focusing decisions on the public's needs.

References

1   Heller T. D., Heller R. F., Pattison S., Fletcher R. Treating the patient or the population? Part 1. Judging the benefit of treatment of individual patients. *West J. Med.* 2001; **175**: 35–7.

2   Heller T. D., Heller R. F., Pattison S., Fletcher R. Treating the patient or the population? Part 2. Judging the benefit of a treatment to society as a whole. *West J. Med.* 2001; **175**: 104–7.

3   Dolan P., Cookson R., Ferguson B. Effect of discussion and deliberation on the public's views of priority setting in health care: focus group study. *BMJ* 1999; **318**: 916–19.

4   Heller R. F., Heller T. D., Pattison S. Putting the public back into public health. Part I. A re-definition of public health. *Public Health* 2003; **117**: 62–5.

5   Heller R. F., Heller T. D., Pattison S. Putting the public back into public health. Part II. How can public health be accountable to the public? *Public Health* 2003; **117**: 66–71.

6   Murray S. A. Experiences with 'rapid appraisal' in primary care: involving the public in assessing health needs, orientating staff, and educating medical students. *BMJ* 1999; **318**: 440–4.

Chapter 12

Evidence into action: population impact assessment and population health decision support

This chapter introduces practical tools to provide support for population health decision-making. In the process, it brings together a number of the themes presented elsewhere in the book.

One of the major impediments to the practice of evidence-based health care has been that the focus has been on collecting and reviewing the evidence rather than on its implementation. Knowing that an intervention leads to a certain relative risk reduction, for example, does not tell us how to translate this into numbers of lives saved, or outcomes prevented, in a particular local population. Nor does it tell us how to prioritize the introduction of this intervention in competition with other alternative interventions or current use of funds. Nor does it tell us what the effect of the intervention on health inequalities will be in the population into which it is to be introduced.

In the field of evidence-based medicine, this issue has been identified, and some measures have been taken to help with implementation. Clinical decision support tools have been developed for use at the point of care.[1] However, in neither the individual nor population health fields is there currently available a means to project the risk reductions identified from systematic reviews to a local population.

I describe two linked attempts to help the policy-maker. First, to help make the measures of the impact of a risk factor or an intervention on the health of the population, *population impact assessment*. Second, to help put the results of this into practice, some *population health decision support* tools. Together, these are designed to produce a set of methods and toolkits that will help public health practitioners and policy-makers to implement the results of trials, systematic reviews of trials and other data on benefits and risks in their populations, to produce localized evidence that can feed directly into decision-making processes.

Population impact assessment

The steps are as follows: It will come as no surprise to the reader that I propose using the Population Health Evidence Cycle[2] as a framework and population impact measures to describe the population impact.

The framework: the Population Health Evidence Cycle

The steps

+ **Ask.** Identify the need and ask the question. Let us take three examples. First, in the UK in 2004, a new contract was introduced for general practitioners. This provided incentives to improve practice whereby financial rewards were to be given for meeting certain practice targets. We looked to see what impact this would make on reducing the burden of deaths from heart disease. We asked the question:

"What is the likely benefit to a typical general practice, expressed as numbers of deaths postponed in the next five years, of going from current practice to the implementation of the new GP contract in terms of cardiovascular disease (CVD) interventions?[3]"

Second, a primary care organisation wishes to increase the level of child immunization in its community. It asks the question:

"What is the impact of increasing measles vaccination from current levels to 100 per cent coverage, in terms of reduced child mortality?"

Third, as part of the exploration of the impact of health inequalities in the UK, and efforts to reduce them, cigarette smoking has emerged as an important cause of health inequality. Answering the question

"What is the number of deaths you might expect in a typical UK General Practice from cigarette smoking among manual and non-manual workers?"

may help identify the priorities for targeting health promotion activities.

- **Collect.** This involves *collecting* all the data required to *calculate* population impact measures (see Chapter 4 for more detail).

- **Understand.** Present data in a clear, understandable and relevant way. You may wish to rank alternative interventions: by numbers of outcome events prevented, numbers prevented per unit cost or cost per number prevented.

- **Use.** Feed into decision-making process and implement change. As we have shown in Chapter 7, the theory of knowledge management can help with the implementation and use of evidence. Having 'generated' knowledge of the population impact numbers is not going to be enough to ensure that they are used appropriately. Storage, distribution and application of knowledge will also be essential, as will the understanding of how to relate the newly derived explicit knowledge to the pre-existing tacit knowledge.

Population health decision support

Although the steps described above seem reasonably simple, the data may be difficult to obtain and help will be required with the calculations so that they can be demystified and used readily in practice.

My colleagues and I plan to develop a set of web-based tools to help the policy-maker obtain the data required for the calculations of population impact measures in their population. This will require help with identifying their population denominator, obtaining published data on baseline risk of the outcome of interest (such as death or hospital readmission) and the relative risks (RR) or relative risk reductions (RRRs) associated with the risk or intervention of interest. The calculation of population impact measures will require data on current local risk factor prevalence or practice levels as well as the goals for risk factor reduction or best practice levels for the use of the intervention in question. Where these are not available locally, we will identify sources for their estimates from similar populations.

The tools will be web-based, will offer links to public health data repositories such as Public Health Observatories (at least for the UK), and will develop libraries of common RRs and RRRs.

The system in operation

The first set of examples shows how to implement population impact assessment for three different types of question. The second two examples will show what the population health decision support system might look like in operation.

Example 1

Introduction of the new GP contract in the UK

- **Ask** the question: "What is the likely benefit to a typical general practice, expressed as numbers of deaths postponed in the next 5 years, of going from current practice to the implementation of the new GP contract in terms of cardiovascular disease (CVD) interventions?"
- **Collect** the data and **calculate** population impact measures.

Population size and composition

You work in a UK General Practice with 10,000 patients on your list, which has the same age and gender distribution as the whole of England and Wales.

Outcome

We will choose death in the next five years as the outcome of interest. The RRRs are taken from recent reviews and are summarized in the table in the paper in which these calculations are published.

Baseline risk

Data from the Framingham Study were used to estimate the five-year CHD event rate. Since we do not have data of our own population, we have had to use data from another population. It is likely that the Framingham event rates exaggerate those in the UK,[4] and this does emphasize the importance of collecting locally relevant data on health outcomes.

Proportion of your population exposed

We can identify current treatment levels from a variety of sources. Best would be to use disease registers which are currently requirements for Primary Care Trusts to maintain as part of the UK Coronary Heart Disease National Service Framework. A number of pieces of relevant information are difficult to obtain from the published literature, such as the way in which drug treatments are combined in individuals, and a goal for future data capture exercises will be to ensure that information necessary for the calculation of population impact measures are actually collected. The estimates used in this calculation are also shown in the paper on which these estimates are based.[5]

Best practice goal

The GP contract defined treatment goals in terms of percentage of the population who should be offered the various interventions—these are also shown in the paper from which this example is drawn.[5]

Time over which outcome is to be assessed

We have defined this as five years. This choice is pragmatic and depends on the availability of data on baseline risk and elative risk reductions from the interventions. Many policy decisions are made over a three-year planning cycle, so we could have used three years instead, if we could obtain the relevant data.

Cost of introducing intervention

I am not presenting economic analyses here. At its simplest level, we would need to examine drug costs of each of the interventions. If we were to calculate the full costs of the intervention, we would have to include a range of expenses, such as doctor and nurse time.

The calculation

The calculation of Number of Events Prevented in this Population of 10,000 people (NEPP) is in Appendix A at the end of this chapter.

Going from current to best practice to meet the contract targets among this population would prevent 57 events over the next five years.

Understand

Presentation of the information in an understandable way is essential. I have taken this from the abstract of the paper, which describes the calculations.[5]

> The greatest health gain, among those aged between 45 and 84 years, would come from reaching cholesterol reduction targets. This could prevent 15, 7 and 7 events among those with raised cholesterol and coronary heart disease, stroke and diabetes respectively. Achieving blood pressure control targets among those with uncontrolled hypertension but without the above conditions could prevent 15 cardiovascular events, with further benefits from reducing blood pressure in patients with high blood pressure and coronary heart disease, stroke or diabetes. Achieving other targets would have smaller impacts, because high levels of care are already being achieved, or because of the lower prevalence of conditions or risk of adverse events.

Use the results

Each GP in the UK should find this information of use, as they decide how to meet the requirements of the GP contract in a way that will maximize the health gain (as well as the financial gain) of implementing the contract.

Example 2

Measles vaccination

- **Ask.** I have set this question in terms of its relevance to a low–middle income country, as: "What is the impact of increasing measles vaccination from current levels to 100 per cent coverage, in terms of reduced infant mortality in the population?"

- **Collect and calculate.** For this, we will calculate a slightly different population impact measure—which uses the attack rate, the vaccine efficiency, the population coverage of the vaccine programme and the cost of the programme[6].

Population size and composition

You work in rural India, with responsibility for the rural health services in an area similar to that of Ballabgarh, with a population size of 74,007 where a study into measles vaccine was performed.[8] We will take a population of 100,000 of whom approximately 11% might be aged 12–60 months (WHO life tables for India).

Outcome

We will choose death in the next year as the outcome of interest. The benefit depends on the Vaccine Efficiency (VE)—which is the vaccination equivalent of the RRR—expressed in relation to the outcome of interest. For measles, this would include morbidity, hospitalization, and infant deaths. A recent review suggests a vaccine efficiency against death (total mortality) of 49 per cent.[7]

Baseline risk

Annual death rates in Indian children aged 12–60 months approximate 10/1,000 (WHO life Tables for India) and we have used 20/1,000 over 2 years.

Proportion of your population exposed

Assume that 56 per cent of children currently receive measles vaccination.[9]

Best practice goal

In Bangladesh 95 per cent of children receive measles vaccine,[9] so this is an appropriate goal.

Time over which outcome is to be assessed

We have defined this as two years. This choice is pragmatic, although the paper used for the source of much of this calculation finds that the impact of vaccination on deaths persists for this time[7].

Cost of introducing intervention

A number of economic evaluations of measles vaccination programmes have been published. I am not going to consider this further here.

The calculation

The calculation of Number of Events Prevented in your Population (NEPP) is given in Appendix B at the end of this chapter.

Understand

The calculations reveal that it is necessary to vaccinate 102 children to prevent a death in the next two years. Among a population of 100,000 children aged 12–60 months, the improvement in measles vaccination from the current 56 per cent to 95 per cent would result in 42 fewer deaths in the next two years.

Use

Once the costs of the vaccination programme have been calculated, this will help the policy-maker decide how much priority to give to improving measles vaccination rates in such a population. The calculation of costs in not easy, and will depend on whether to go for catch-up vaccination in the whole age group at risk or to focus on vaccinating those reaching the appropriate vaccination age for the first time. A full cost-effectiveness estimate might be required for this level of detail, but the need to target measles vaccination in such a population is very clear from the demonstration of these figures.

Example 3

Calculation of the population burden of risk of cigarette smoking

- ◆ **Ask.** "What is the number of deaths you might expect in a typical UK General Practice from cigarette smoking among manual and non-manual men?" Answering this question will help identify the priorities for targeting health promotion activities in your population.

◆ **Collect and calculate.** For this, we will calculate 'PIN-ER-*t*' or The Population Impact Number of Eliminating a Risk factor, defined as "the potential number of disease events prevented in your population over the next t years by eliminating a risk factor."[1] See Appendix C at the end of this chapter.

Population size and composition

Again, we will use a typical UK General Practice population of 10,000 people. With some assumptions, there would be 1589 and 1810 men aged 25 years or more in non-manual and manual groups respectively among such a population.

Outcome

The relative risk of death from smoking is estimated to be the same in manual and non-manual groups and to be 2.19.

Baseline risk

For the first application, we have taken the annual risk of death from any cause in men having either manual or non-manual occupations from data supplied to us by the Office for National Statistics (ONS) as described in a previous publication.[10]

Proportion of your population exposed

The prevalence of cigarette smoking in manual and non-manual groups (33 per cent and 22 per cent respectively) was taken from the 2001 *General Household Survey.*[11]

Time over which outcome is to be assessed

The time period *(t)* over which the consequences of a risk factor are being considered is important in the process of allocating resources for relevant treatment or prevention services. Most current reviews of health service resource in the UK take place in three-yearly cycles; therefore we have used PIN-ER-3 for the examples in this paper.

The calculation

The calculation reveals that over the next three years, there will be 5 and 13 deaths respectively among non-manual and manual men in this population as a result of cigarette smoking.

Table 12.1 Calculation of Population Impact Numbers for Population Impact Assessment

Issue	Population size abd target groups	Proportion with the condition (P_d)	Baseline risk of outcome and time over which assessed	Proportion of population currently treated	Best practice goal	Relative Risk Reduction or Relative Risk	Population impact
GP contract in UK	10,000 practice population: 3144 aged 45–84	~10% have heart disease	~15% have CVD event in 5 years	Varies according to intervention	See Table 7.1, p 70	Varies according to intervention	57 cardiovascular events prevented in next 5 years
Measles vaccination in India	100,000 population: Assume 11,000 aged 12–59 months	N/A, total population impact	20/1000 deaths in next 2 years	56% vaccinated	95%	49%	42 deaths prevented by vaccination in next 2 years
Smoking and social class	10,000 practice population: 1589 'non-manual' and 1810 'manual' men aged 25+ years	N/A, total population impact	1.6% of 'non-manual'; 2.5% of 'manual': dead in next 3 years	22% non-manual 33% manual current smoker	N/A, looking at risk	2.19	5 'non-manual'; 13 'manual' deaths in next 3 years from smoking

Note: Many of the estimates may not be accurate, and a sensitivity analysis using a range of alternative estimates should be performed.

Understand

The presentation of these numbers will allow a policy-maker to appreciate the burden of illness from cigarette smoking in the context of social inequalities in health risk behaviour.

Use

The policy-maker can now explore the potential costs and benefits of interventions aimed at different sections of the population, and prioritize such interventions against alternative uses of funds and alternative benefits.

Box 12.1 Components of population impact assessment

Ask the question—make the options explicit

Collect data—local data on population denominator/prevalence and current practice (or published data from similar populations)/ estimated data on baseline risk of identified outcomes (from Observatory etc)/library of evidence for risks (Relative Risk and Relative Risk Reduction).

Calculate impact—population impact measures or alternatives

Understand—apply values, offer training, consultation

Use—implement results in prioritising services using change management and knowledge management (generate, store, distribute and apply).

Population health decision support— what it might look like

Although the system is not fully developed, these are the steps and the help that might be available to support the decision-making process.

Step 1: Measure the population impact

(A) Impact of a risk factor

1 Define the decision you want to make—**Ask** the question.

2 **Collect** the data you require:

- What is the size of the population to which the decision refers?

- What is the outcome you want to examine, as defined in your question? This might be deaths, hospital admissions, cost-effectiveness etc.

- What is the baseline risk of this outcome in your population? How to find this: assuming you do not have data available in your own population, first try the Public Health Observatory web site (www.pho.org.uk). Make sure you define the length of time over which you want to examine the outcome—such as one year or three years.

- What is the prevalence of the risk factor in your population? If you do not have access to local data, go to a national database for data which you might be able to use. In the UK, the Health Survey for England and Wales offers a large amount of data.

- What is the RR of the outcome you have chosen in the presence of the risk factor of interest? A single source for relative risks for common risk factors does not currently exist—this will be an early task for the development of the population health decision support system. In the meantime, a literature search will probably be required.

3 **Calculate** the population impact measure—for a risk factor the PIN-ER-t will be most useful. A web based calculator already exists in an early form http://simph.man.ac.uk.

Or:

(B) Impact of an intervention

1 Define the decision you want to make—**Ask** the question.

2 **Collect** the data you require:

- What is the size of the population to which the decision refers? (To keep this simple in the examples, we will only consider a single population rather than a set of subpopulations defined by age, gender, ethnicity or deprivation—refined versions of this will allow these distributions to be entered and allowed for in the calculations.)

- What is the outcome you want to examine, as defined in your question? This might be deaths, hospital admissions, cost-effectiveness etc.

- What is the baseline risk of this outcome in your population? How to find this:assuming you do not have data available in your own population, first try the Public Health Observatory web site (http://www.pho.org.uk). Make sure you define the length of time over which you want to examine the outcome—such as one year or three years.

- What is the current practice level of use of the intervention in question in your population? If you do not have access to local data such as audit or survey data, go to a national database for data which you might be able to use. This is likely to require a literature search.

- What is the best practice goal which you wish to achieve? This may come from guidelines or local consensus or national targets.

- What is the RRR of the outcome you have chosen in response to the introduction of the intervention of interest? A single source for relative risk reductions for common interventions does not currently exist—this will be an early task for the development of the population health decision support system. In the meantime, a literature search will probably be required. Access to relevant web sites such as the Cochrane Collaboration's Health Promotion and Public Health Field, http://www.vichealth.vic.gov.au/cochrane/ and Guide to Community Preventive Services http://www.thecommunityguide.org will be provided.

3 **Calculate** the population impact measure—the NEPP may be the most useful. A web-based simulator does not currently exist as it does for the PIN-ER-t, although one is under construction.

Now, having measured the impact, complete the task of implementing the results.

Step 2: Understand the population impact

This requires that the results are presented in a way that can be appreciated by those who will be responsible for implementing the decision. Two tasks are required—first education about the measures used, their derivation and meaning. This will be helped by educational resources linked to a population health decision support web site—at each stage an explanation of all terms and calculations will be provided. Second, a simple presentation format for the results of the impact assessment will be developed. Until these are developed, readers of this book, or those who have learnt the skills through the online MPHe course (http://www.mphe.man.ac.uk) will be able to act as advisors to those who want to use the methods.

Step 3: Use the information by feeding into the decision-making process and manage the change required for the implementation

This will require an appreciation of the implicit knowledge held by those responsible for the implementation, and how the new explicit knowledge can be shown to add to it. The support system will ask:

◆ What are the current drivers of the service provision?

◆ Have you identified the interest served by not adopting change?

◆ Have you identified the costs of change and no change?

◆ Have you identified the implicit knowledge of those responsible for the implementation, and how this might be changed by the presentation of the new explicit knowledge obtained through the population impact assessment?

Step 4: Evaluate the change introduced and attempt to measure the benefits of the decision

This may necessitate a return to Step 1 of this process (Ask the question) and require another run through the system.

Key summary points

◆ *The Student.* Use of the Population Health Evidence Cycle will offer help to the policy-maker in prioritizing between alternative uses of resource to ease the population burden of illness.

◆ *The Practitioner.* Population impact assessment can be useful in order to calculate and present the impact in your population of both risks and benefits. The use of local data is seen to be essential to this, and emphasizes the importance of collecting local data on baseline risk, disease and risk factor prevalence and current practice levels.

◆ *The Policy-maker*. The population health decision support systems presented here should be of use in prioritizing between alternative uses of resource. Despite the existence of, and need for, more complex measures of cost-effectiveness, access to web-based decision support systems into which local data may be fed should make a contribution to health policy-making. Use of the decision support systems should be based on principles of knowledge management— storage, distribution and application of the information generated.

Box 12.2 Components of population health decision support

◆ Provide web-based decision support system

◆ Provide access to each component of the population impact assessment

◆ Provide tools to calculate population impact measures

◆ Provide online training to use and understand results

◆ Provide simple presentation of results

◆ Provide schema for change management to implement results

Appendix A. Example 1: Introduction of the new GP contract in the UK

Number of Events Prevented in your Population (NEPP) = Population size $*$ $P_e * P_d *$ Baseline risk $*$ RRR where P_e is the proportion of the diseased population eligible for treatment (shorthand for the difference between prevalence of current treatment levels and best practice) and P_d is the proportion of the population with the disease.

Sample calculation for aspirin: Among a UK population of 10,000 people, there would be 1154 men aged 45–64, 8.365 per cent of whom have heart disease (P_d), and they have a five-year risk of a cardiovascular event of 12.8 per cent. Of these men, 81 per cent are already on treatment with aspirin, and the target being 90 per cent (of the 90 per cent without contraindications to aspirin). The RRR from the use of aspirin is 25 per cent:

$$NEPP = 1154*0.08365*(0.9*(0.9–0.81))*0.128*0.25 = 0.25.$$

Thus increasing aspirin use will have little impact; a quarter of an event saved over 5 years. For all cardiovascular interventions in the contract, 57 events would be prevented.

Appendix B. Example 2: Measles vaccination

We are going to calculate the Number needed to vaccinate to prevent one event (NNV) 1/(Death rate × Vaccine effectiveness) and the Number needed to target to prevent one event (NTV) (which takes into account the proportion of the population who currently receive and who should receive vaccination).[6] 1/(Death rate × Vaccine effectiveness) × (target proportion to be vaccinated − proportion of population currently vaccinated). In order to relate this to a particular population, we will calculate the number of events prevented in your population (NEPP) = population size/NTV:

$$NNV = 1/0.02 \times 0.49 = 102$$
$$NTV = 1/0.02 \times 0.49 \times 0.39 = 261.6$$
$$NEPP \text{ from vaccination} = 100000/61.6 = 42$$

Thus 42 deaths prevented in a population of 100,000 children.

Appendix C. Example 3: Cigarette smoking

The full formula for PIN-ER-t is:

$$N * I_p * [P_e(RR − 1)/ 1 + P_e(RR − 1)] \quad or \quad N * I_p * PAR$$

Where N is the population size, I_p is the three-year death rate and P_e is the prevalence of smoking in that population, RR is the relative risk of death from smoking, and PAR is Population Attributable Risk—see Chapter 4.

Details of the calculation among non-manual men:

$$[P_e(RR − 1)/ 1 + P_e(RR − 1)] = 0.22 * (2.19−1)/1$$
$$+ 2.19 * (2.19−1) = 0.21$$

(i.e. 21 per cent of the total mortality among non-manual men over the next three years is due to their smoking.)

PIN-ER-3   or   N * I_p * [PAR]: 1589 * 0.016069 * 0.21 = 5.10

(i.e. five deaths in non-manual men in that population over the next three years will be due to cigarette smoking.)

References

1 O'Connor A. M., Legare F., Stacey D. Risk communication in practice: the contribution of decision aids. *BMJ* 2003; **327**: 736–40.

2 Heller R. F., Heller T. D., Pattison S. Putting the public back into public health. Part II. How can public health be accountable to the public? *Public Health* 2003; **117**: 66–71.

3 McElduff P., Lyratzopoulos G., Edwards R., Heller R. F., Shekelle P., Roland M. Will changes in primary care improve health outcomes? Modelling the impact of financial incentives introduced to improve quality of care in the UK. *Qual Saf Health Care* 2004; **13**: 191–7.

4 Brindle P., Emberson J., Lampe F., Walker M., Whincup P., Fahey T., *et al.* Predictive accuracy of the Framingham coronary risk score in British men: prospective cohort study. *BMJ* 2003; **327**: 1267.

5 McElduff P., Lyratzopoulos G., Edwards R., Heller R. F., Shekelle P., Roland M. Will changes in primary care improve health outcomes? Modelling the impact of financial incentives introduced to improve quality of care in the UK. *Qual.Saf Health Care* 2004; **13**: 191–7.

6 Kelly H., Attia J., Andrews R., Heller R. F. The number needed to vaccinate (NNV) and population extensions of the NNV: comparison of influenza and pneumococcal vaccine programmes for people aged 65 years and over. *Vaccine* 2004; **22**: 2192–8.

7 Aaby P., Bhuiya A., Nahar L., Knudsen K., de Francisco A., Strong M. The survival benefit of measles immunization may not be explained entirely by the prevention of measles disease: a community study from rural Bangladesh. *Int. J. Epidemiol.* 2003; **32**: 106–16.

8 Kabir Z., Long J., Reddaiah V. P., Kevany J., Kapoor S. K. Non-specific effect of measles vaccination on overall child mortality in an area of rural India with high vaccination coverage: a population-based case-control study. *Bull. World Health Organ* 2003; **81**: 244–50.

9 Zaidi A. K., Awasthi S., deSilva H. J. Burden of infectious diseases in South Asia. *BMJ* 2004; **328**: 811–15.

10 Heller R. F., Buchan I., Edwards R., Lyratzopoulos G., McElduff P., St Leger S. Communicating risks at the population level: application of population impact numbers. *BMJ* 2003; **327**: 1162–5.

11 Walker A., O'Brien M., Traynor J., Fox K., Goddard E., Foster, K. *Living in Britain 2001: Health Survey for England 2001*. London, The Stationery Office: Office for National Statistics, 2002.

Index